Crystal Power:
Mythology and History

Crystal Power

Mythology and History

The Mystery, Magic and Healing Properties
of Crystals, Stones and Gems

Andreas Guhr
Jörg Nagler

Foreword by Michael Gienger

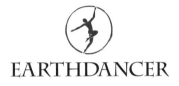

EARTHDANCER

A FINDHORN PRESS IMPRINT

Publisher's Note

All the information in this book has been compiled according to the publisher's best knowledge and belief. People react in different ways, however, so that neither the publisher, nor the author can, in individual cases, provide a guarantee for the effectiveness or harmlessness of the applications described herein. In cases of serious health problems or mental problems please consult a physician, alternative practitioner or psychologist.

1 2 3 4 5 6 7 20 19 18 17 16 15 14 13 12 11 10 09 08 07 06

Andreas Guhr and Jörg Nagler
Crystal Power: Mythology and History

Copyright © Neue Erde GmbH/Andreas Guhr
First published in Germany in 1995 by Ellert & Richter, Hamburg as *Mythos der Steine*

This English edition © 2006 Earthdancer GmbH
English translation © 2006 Astrid Mick

Title cover: Dragon Design, UK
Edited by Stuart Booth
Typeset in ITC Garamond Condensed

Published by Earthdancer Books, an Imprint of:
Findhorn Press, 305a The Park, Findhorn, Forres IV36 3TE, Great Britain

Printed in China

ISBN 10 = 1-84409-085-X
ISBN 13 = 978-1-84409-085-3

Contents

The Roots
of Crystal Healing
Michael Gienger

Some 20 years since its first publication, *Myths of Crystals* has become a standard reference work gaining in regard year by year. The book provides a clear, understandable description of the roots of crystal healing, which is now on the cusp of being recognised as a valid naturopathic treatment. Whilst 20 years ago healing with crystals was known to "initiated circles" only, nowadays it can no longer be dismissed from naturopathy. This is all the more reason therefore to become familiar with its roots and ancient origins.

The ancient tradition of crystal healing is still an important source for a full understanding and appreciation of the nature and effects of crystals and gems. Its ancient tradition is the essence of experience gained over a very long period of time. As such, that healing tradition is one of an ongoing encounter and interaction between humans and stone – and what happens during these encounters.

The role of crystals, stones and gems has been central to many pictures, myths and legends. Quite often, the name of the crystal or gem is itself actually derived from a myth. For example: "amethyst" is the "one who is not drunk" (from the Greek amethyein, "to safeguard against drunkenness"); "diamond" is the "invincible one" (from the same meaning in Greek, adamas); "haematite" is the "blood stone" (Greek haemateios, "bloody"); and there are many more.

Modern research into crystal healing is barely twenty years old, so the treasury of knowledge concealed in the myths about crystals and gems is a particularly valuable resource. Many of the properties and healing effects of crystals that have been handed down have turned out to be confirmed in modern practice.

For this reason, it is advisable for all those who work with crystal healing – whether as laymen or therapists – to know something about the roots of the old traditions.

In such a context this is, then, a particularly important book, as it gives a detailed, historical account of the best-known myths and legends surrounding crystals, gems and stones. Unfortunately, there appear to be too many authors nowadays who invent myths purposely in order to support their own (often spurious) work of similarly invented and alleged effects of the crystals with their manufactured "pseudo-histories". The Tiger's Eye for example, did not arrive in Europe from South Africa until the nineteenth century, yet was mentioned in connection with Arab and classical Greek traditions.

This is where the book becomes a great help in "separating the wheat from the chaff". It has been correctly, scientifically researched and all the sources verified – so that it also debunks those phoney myths and any associated and dubious crystal properties.

I venture to say that you hold in your hands a book that is a truly valuable asset for all who love crystals and stones and actually use them. Realistically, it is only through direct personal encounters and experiences with crystals that one will truly understand the traditions collected and presented here. Nevertheless, this book will open an extra world of knowledge, providing the reader with the important heritage of our long history and cultural relationship with stones, gems and crystals – maybe long forgotten, but now once again at our disposal and for our benefit.

Michael Gienger
Tübingen, Spring 2005

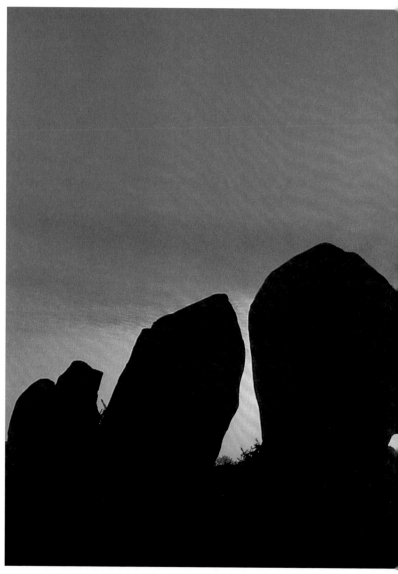

What is often termed "The "Riddle of Carnac" in Brittany has never been solved. Thousands of granite monoliths stand in the landscape

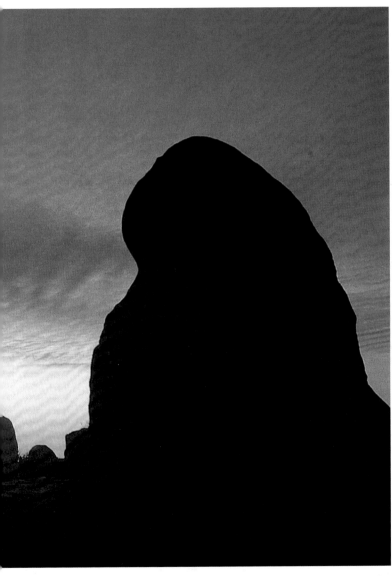

*row upon row, bearing witness to a highly developed culture around
3000BC. Some of these stones weigh more than 350 tonnes.*

From Stones to Gems

From the beginning of the Palaeolithic period, or Old Stone Age (about 300,000 to 100,000 BC), our ancestors adopted a hunter gatherer lifestyle. Stones with sharp edges, which could be shaped into tools, hand axes, and stone blades, made it possible to overcome a relative physical weaknesses and also to shape the environment to a much greater degree than ever before. This adoption of stone, with its pre-eminent importance in both use and function, was a process that took hundreds of thousands of years. Nevertheless, it resulted in humans incorporating stone into religions and thereby conferring stone with outstandingly important significance. Even the early peoples of the Palaeolithic period tried to enlist the help of stones through the medium of scratching magical symbols and thereby bestowing certain meanings on the stones carrying such markings – and all this long, long before the existence of even the first rudiments of writing.

Consequently, a magic, holy or sacred stone was a ritual object. Heaps of stones, such as cairns, indicated the location of sites of worship. Stone balls from the Palaeolithic Mousterian period (named after their find site, Le Moustier in the Dordogne region of France) have been dated to between 150,000 and 60,000 BC. They are probably some of the first known evidence of such cult sites and may well be interpreted as symbols of the Sun. Here, for the first time, something emerged in human history that was not immediately connected with survival. Stone balls similar to these have also been found in the Charente region of western French and in North Africa.

The notion that stone is the seat of the divine can also be found in many later religions. The sacred stone of the Canaanite religion was called bethel, meaning "house of God", and gave the name to the village mentioned in the New Testament as well as being within the name of Bethlehem. Additionally in Christianity, Jesus appears as the "corner stone" and the community of the Church" as "living stones".

If a stone is seen as the "House of God", then it is not so large a step to a stone altar on which sacrificial offerings are made to the god(s). Stone as the "House of God" functioned as "the protective", "the giver of fertility",

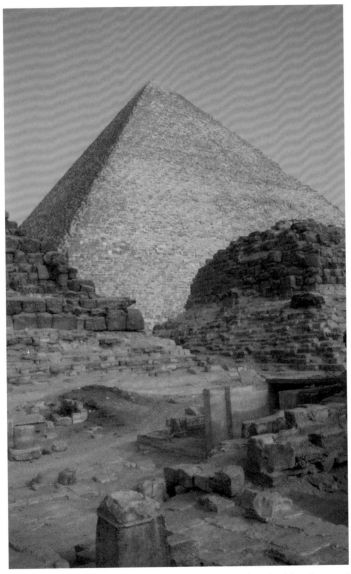

The pyramids – five-thousand-year-old symbols of the highly advanced civilisation of Ancient Egypt.

"the immortal". Its durability allowed it to become the most important element of a cult of death. The presence of stone was intended to ensure eternal existence, but also prevent access to the world of the living by the inhabitants of the kingdom of the dead. From a simple stone tomb to the pyramid – all these manifestations of stone are based on this idea about stone. Our present-day tombstones serve to keep alive our remembrance of the dead for generations to come.

In Neolithic western Europe (c. 5000 to 2000 BC), there was a spread of cultures that were characterised by sites of worship with megaliths structures that represent the best known of all evidence of the veneration of stones and their use: Dolmens and menhirs (chamber tombs made of stone arranged in a table-like fashion), passage graves, roofed tombs and the stone rows of Carnac in Brittany, which are 200 to 1500m (656 to 4,921ft). Finally, there is one of the most impressive sites of all, the gigantic stone circle of Stonehenge in southern England, which presumably also served as a means for astronomical calculations.

Further Neolithic finds in south-western England are the two famous holed stones of Men-an-Tol at Madron, in Cornwall. The openings in the centres of these stones have diameters of 40cm (16 inches) and 53cm (21 inches), respectively and it is assumed that sick children were passed through the holes for healing purposes, to quasi ("strip off") their illness. This is only one of the many example showing how deeply rooted were the ancient peoples' ideas, about the healing effect of stones.

Where naturally occurring formations of holes in stones or rock were present – often caused by inclusions of sedimentary fossils or other types of rock – they were always considered to be something magical. The use of stones in this way goes back to the Palaeolithic period, from which there have been finds of stone beads used for necklaces, etc. Later, with the evolution of more advanced cultures and their associated, improved technologies, humans managed to drill holes in stones themselves. This was an important step, as it then became possible to create jewellery deliberately for body decoration and even place stones in settings. So was born the amulet made of stone and crystal.

Carnelian is the only gemstone which we are certain was worked during the Mesolithic (Middle Stone Age) being made into the most delicate, sharp blades in the region of Durddanskayaand Akcha in Siberia. In some prehistoric tombs, carnelian was also found in the shape of tiny balls with holes drilled through them, i.e. for use as beads. The possession of such beads must have been of great importance and may well have contributed to the warding off of evil spirits.

Sumeria

> "O ye gods here present!
> Just as surely as I shall not forget
> This lapis lazuli upon my neck,
> So I shall remember these days,
> Never forgetting them."
> The Epic of Gilgamesh

The Sumerians, whose origins are still unknown, settled in Mesopotamia, the "land between the rivers" Euphrates and Tigris. As early as the fourth millennium BC, they were familiar with the art of working precious stones and gems. They had already used them as "miracle stones", which were imbued, so they believed, with magical powers. So, here already is a belief in the healing powers of crystals and stones. Some of them were believed to be effective against illnesses, others were used for love problems, and others even to protect the owner or wearer from thieves. The cylindrical seals that were in use in Mesopotamia from about 3300 BC and which had replaced stamp seals, were made out of crystals such as lapis lazuli, serpentine and haematite. They were used for sealing the storage chambers in the temple precinct, with different sized seals being given to the different dignitaries. The gods were provided with cylinder seals with lengths of up to 16 cm (just over 6 inches); a prince, by contrast, could only claim a seal with a size of about 6cm (about $2\,^1/_2$ inches). Archaeological digs gradually

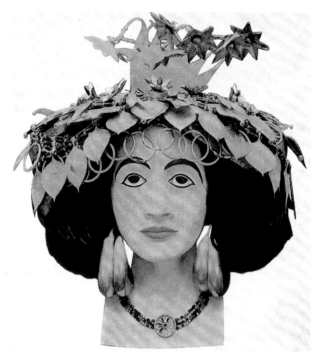

Reconstruction of the golden headdress of the Sumerian Queen Shub-A, who died in about 2700 BC.

brought to light countless such cylinder seals. Since most of them were made out of precious stones, it is justifiable to assume that crystals and gemstones were in everyday use in Mesopotamia - at least for members of the upper classes. The Assyriologist Samuel Noah Kramer has described some of these seals as follows: "One of the favourite subjects for gem cutters in southern Mesopotamia was a scene in which a man is introduced to one god by another god; probably the owner of the seal was being introduced to his personal patron divinity. Further north, in Assyria, the gem cutters developed an entire repertoire of objects and styles with heraldic motifs, animal fight scenes and stories about the gods."

In order to drill a hole in these seals, which were of great value to the owners, the Sumerians employed drilling tools that made it possible to work even the harder types of gem. The seals were threaded on a string, either lengthwise or may have been carried on the owner's belt. Thus was taken the next step in manufacturing jewellery.

The famous royal tombs, which were uncovered in 1922 in the ruins of the ancient city of Ur at Sumer, also yielded gems of the most beautiful workmanship. In a total of sixteen burial installations of the kings and princesses or priestesses, among the grave offerings were found pieces of jewellery of great perfection. Also found were the remains of other burials, such as of guards and ladies-in-waiting, who had accompanied the King and the priestesses in death – voluntarily or otherwise! C. W. Ceram described one of these finds in more detail: "On a thickly padded wig were found lined up three strings of lapis lazuli and red carnelian. The lowest one had golden rings hanging from it, the second had gold beech leaves, and the third had willow leaves and golden flowers. Above these, a comb with five teeth had been inserted; it was decorated with golden flowers and lapis lazuli."

As a gaming board found in the royal tombs demonstrates, items of the royal inventory were also decorated with precious gems. Sumerian inscriptions contain numerous names of gems, which can be connected with this find and other similar ones. For example, the golden robes of statues of gods, as of the creator and sun god, Marduk of Babylon, were inlaid with precious gems.

As is known from the excavations of the royal tombs of Ur, in addition to the obligatory linen strips for the royal interments, precious gems were also enclosed. Later, gems were also used in architecture. Thus, King Nebuchadnezzar had the roof of the temple at Borsippa decorated with gold and precious gems. Jasper was one of the decorative stones most used by the Sumerians. It was employed both as a material for carving figures of the gods, as well as for protective and healing purposes. Pregnant women often used jasper in order to ease their pregnancy and labour.

Other much-used gems were the midnight blue, gold-flecked lapis lazuli, the delicately coloured beryl, the green emerald, and the diamond. The Cassite kings (sixteenth to twelfth centuries BC), used lapis lazuli as an important trade item to exchange with Egypt for gold. Green malachite was also very popular and a piece of this mineral was found in the form of a tiny bag, among others items of grave goods, in the vault of a Babylonian queen.

In surviving literary inscriptions from the Sumerians – for example, in the *Epic of Gilgamesh*, which was recorded about 1200 BC – crystals and gems are mentioned on a number of occasions. Thus, Gilgamesh is looking for the "precious gem trees" of the garden of the gods:
"Upon seeing the bejewelled shrubs, he approaches them. The carnelian bears its fruit, And hung it is with goodly vines. The lapis lazuli bears leaves; Lush fruit also hangs from it. It is fine to the eye." The highest-ranking goddess swears by her amulet made of lapis lazuli, and a goldsmith creates an image out of this stone, which turns up again and again in the *Epic of Gilgamesh*; obsidian is also mentioned. Precious stones are also referred to as the material for making precious items of use: "On the horizon there appeared the first intimations of dawn; Gilgamesh ... brought out a large table of elammaqu wood, took a carnelian bowl,filled it with honey,took a lapis lazuli bowl, filled it with milk curd..."

A Sumerian hymn describes a temple that was built entirely out of silver and lapis lazuli and the foundations of which contain red carnelian. Precious stones were also equated with luck and positive forces, both in the literary texts, as well as in the spoken language. The notion that the stars were connected with precious stones and that they could beneficially influence them was also intimately connected with these beliefs. The star cult, in turn, was closely connected with the belief in gods, so that the Sumerian–Babylonian cuneiform symbol for "star" and the ideograph for "God" were identical.

Astrology, which originated in Babylon, tried to decode the constellations among the stars and to fathom their connection with the fate of humans.

Egypt

> "I have taken possession of the Ureret crown;
> Ma'at (i.e., right and truth) is in my body;
> its mouths are of turquoise and rock crystal.
> My homestead is among the furrows
> which are [of the colour of] lapis lazuli."
>
> Egyptian Book of the Dead

This is from the translation by Sir E. A. Wallis Budge of the Ancient Egyptian *Book of the Dead*, based on various papyri (including the Papyrus of Ani) when he was Keeper of Egyptian and Assyrian Antiquities at the British Museum, and first published 1899.

The belief in a continuing life after death evolved particularly in ancient Egypt – the "gift of the Nile", as Egypt was referred to by Herodotus. So, there is no real surprise in the many references to crystals and gems in the Egyptian *Book of the Dead*. To the Ancient Egyptians, these gems and stones symbolised all that was immortal – things that would not lose their beauty or brilliance, even after death. From this belief stemmed the concept that the deceased should be able to move around in pleasant surroundings and feel comfortable in the Otherworld. The clear separation between life and death that is very familiar to us these days was far removed from the Egyptian view of the world. A stone, especially a crystal or precious gem, symbolised the eternal. Thus, it was quite normal to allow any stone or gem, which had already adorned the wearer in his or her lifetime, to accompany him or her as protection and adornment on a path that led into the Unknown.

With their associations and equation with immortality, the use and importance of crystals and gems was part of Egyptian mythology from a very early stage of its development. A particularly interesting aspect of all this is that the considerable number of known types of crystals nevertheless had only a few names in the ancient Egyptian language. One reason may be that all of the main crystals used were merely designated in a few groups by colour – for example, "blue stone", "red stone" and "green stone". Thus, jasper was a "green stone", rock crystal a "white stone", with obsidian and haematite classified as "black stones". Only much later, from the time of the Middle Kingdom onwards, was the term "the violet amethyst" used more often, with its Egyptian name being derived from its Nubian trading centre.

The Ancient Egyptians assigned different "moods", based upon colour, to the most popular crystals and gems. As a result, the word for the "red stone", carnelian, also meant "anger" and "fury". In the same way, the word for the greenish stone, turquoise, equated with "freshness" and "growth". So, if carnelian was replaced with turquoise it was tantamount to driving away anger with joy.

Green gems were the most popular of all in Ancient Egypt. They were reminiscent of the annual greening of the Nile Valley, when the river transformed the dry, brown land into a green oasis, seeming like a miracle. Just as in Sumeria, divine characteristics and features were also described with the use of the names of precious crystals and gems. For instance, this was how Osiris, god of the realm of the dead and brother and husband to the goddess Isis, was praised: "You are the one, who has limbs of gold, a head of lapis lazuli and a crown of turquoise"

Not only gods were compared with and sung about through crystals and gems. The following lines about the beauty of a king's daughter may still be seen on the famous Shabaka Stone from Ancient Egypt, and now housed in the British Museum: "Your charm is like the charm of Anath your beauty is like that of Aschtarat [Astoreth] your hair shimmers like lapis lazuli your eyelid is like unto an onyx bowl, surrounded with rubies."

From the *Book of the Dead* in the chapters from the Papyrus of Ani come the following lines: "Hail to thee, who art full of splendour, Atum Horakhte! When you appear on the horizon... You shine upon the Two Lands with the brilliance of malachite."

Another gemstone connection within ancient Egyptian mythology is in its explanation of how the stars were created. The story goes that a celestial goddess sowed "green stones" in the heavens. Among others, these were

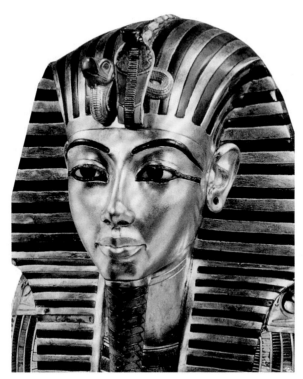

Mummy mask of Pharaoh Tutankhamun (18th dynasty, c.1340 BC) from his tomb in the Valley of the Kings at Thebes. Gold, with inlays of lapis lazuli, turquoise, carnelian, feldspar and paste.

malachite and turquoise. In the *Book of the Dead*, the god of the air, called Shu, planted two turquoise sycamores in the heavens, between which Ra, the Sun, then appears.

The myths that form part of the *Book of the Dead* are a collection of such mythologies, and include sayings that were carved on gems - for example, on jasper, which played an especially important part in the magical glyptics (the art of cutting gems) of the Ancient Egyptians. These sayings were also carved on lapis lazuli, carnelian, serpentine and other types of crystals, precious stones and gems. Using the positions of the Sun and the Moon, it was possible to make exact calculations about when it was most auspicious to carve hieroglyphs into gems. Thus, each extract from the *Book of the Dead* was engraved into a particular type of crystal, and each type was assigned to the appropriate god, who could be invoked in the specific text of the Book.

In fact, many of the gods were identified with celestial bodies and this appears to be the origin of the connection in Ancient Egyptian mythology between the stars and crystals.

The magical sayings or spells that were intended to protect the deceased in the Otherworld and lend him eternal life were to be whispered over golden amulets inlaid with precious gems. His soul was, at the same time, compared with a brilliant gemstone; "Liberate my soul, oh thou Eye of Horus! Like unto a jewel, let it adorn the brow of Ra."

Exact instructions about how to affix a carnelian amulet to the body of a dead person can also be found in the *Book of the Dead*. The deceased was then able to find peace in the "turquoise abodes of the heavens".

The meaning of precious gems and crystals for the Egyptians is most impressively emphasised with a passage from the *Book of the Dead*, in

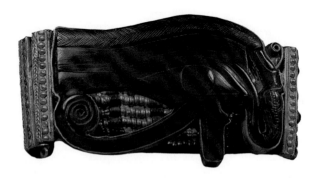

Armband, made of gold, carnelian, fayence and glass from the right lower arm of Tutankhamun's mummy

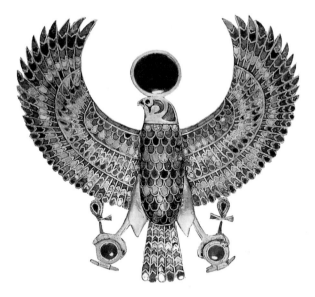

Protective amulet of Pharaoh Tutankhamun made of gold, semi-precious stones and glass.

which a deceased person is addressed, "Your breast is blue like lapis lazuli your locks are darker than the gloomy portals of the house of the dead Ra's rays illuminate your visage your dress woven with gold is decorated with lapis lazuli your limbs, bursting with vigour, covered in gold your breasts swell, like crystal eggs Horus has coloured them with lapis lazuli your shoulders are transparent as crystal."

The grave goods of Tutankhamun, which have now become world-famous, compare very well with these descriptions. The death mask was inlaid with lapis lazuli, carnelian, alabaster and obsidian. His "magical armour" too was covered in amulets made of haematite and carnelian. Tutankhamun was found bedded in a number of layers of gold and jewels when archaeologists first entered the chamber tomb. Howard Carter, the discoverer of this burial site, wrote about the first time he stepped into the actual tomb chamber and how seeing the fabulous treasures actually felt almost like a violation or desecration. Nevertheless, the significance of the find was immediate: "A single glance was enough to convince us that the greatest treasures of the burial were in here."

Most of the items of jewellery in the "treasure chamber" of Tutankhamun had been specially made for the Afterlife. The young king had only worn a few of the rings, amulets and chains in his lifetime. Seven huge pectorals covered the chest and shoulders of the mummy.

They all depict the same figures of creatures with outspread wings made of gold, which form an almost complete semi-circle intended to provide the wearer with magical protection. Turquoise, jasper and carnelian decorate these pectorals, which consequently glow in tones of mainly green and red. The king wears an armband on his right lower arm, the main element of which is formed by a sacred udjat-eye carved out of carnelian. Next to the beetle-based scarab, the udjat-eye was the most popular symbol of Ancient Egypt and was worn as protection against various illnesses, usually against diseases of the eyes. It was also intended to serve the dead as protection, as well as – and this was its main function – to aid with passing through the different regions of the Otherworld. Taking into account the fact that Tutankhamun was a relatively unimportant king, one can imagine what the decorative state of the "eternal abodes" of the important princes must have looked like. Unfortunately, tomb robbers got there long before the archaeologists.

When Tutankhamun was buried in about 1360 BC, the Egyptians were looking back on a tradition of working gems for jewellery that was already some two thousand years old. This is clearly indicated by certain finds with plenty of evidence; for example, drilled stones in the form of the links of a chain.

However, amulets were not only placed in graves and tombs. Rather, the living also used them as protection. Carnelian beads were used for "love magic", and nephrite was intended to protect the wearer from drowning. During the pharaonic period, the scarab is the most prominent among the shaped gems, and served both as an amulet as well as a seal. Amulets kept at the head end of the bed were supposed to bestow peaceful sleep. Both figures and emblems provided models for amulets made of gems; these were, among others, animals, gods and symbols of life. The *Book of the Dead* provides evidence that the type of stone in question definitely determined the intended effect of the item. Heart-shaped amulets, for example, were made out of lapis lazuli, carnelian, or blue-green feldspar; scarabs out of greenstone; and "Isis blood" out of carnelian. It is believed that the alleged magical powers of the gems were derived from the divine origins attributed to them.

Thus, for example, red stones were connected with the blood of the gods, yellow ones with the skin and blue ones with the hair of the gods. The art of the Egyptian goldsmiths was highly developed and influenced the art of jewellery making of antiquity far beyond the pharaonic period. Precious gems were worked into necklaces of beads or set in gold as diadems, armbands, ankle rings or earrings. The stones that the Egyptians required for this work were sourced from their own expeditions – very often from the Sinai Peninsula, where several turquoise mines were to be found. Lapis lazuli was acquired through military expeditions in the regions of Syria and Babylonia. Nubian gems, such as carnelian and amethyst, were sent by the local governor to Egypt as tribute.

The Middle East and Asia Minor

In contrast to the wealth of gems in Egypt and Mesopotamia, artefacts made of gems and crystals were almost completely absent among the Hittites culture of Asia Minor that flourished and developed into a highly sophisticated stage during the second millennium BC. Only haematite seems to have been used, as found in the form of a few seals and as employed among the Hittites for exorcism.

However, in many places ancient Anatolian jewellery made of rock crystal and carnelian has been found dating from the Bronze Age.

In ancient Persia, on the other hand, precious stones were highly prized. In a practice similar to that of the Sumerians and the Egyptians, precious stones were dedicated as valuable burial gifts among the Persians. The most popular were turquoise, lapis lazuli, and carnelian. "Magical" gems were also employed at the ceremony of the consecration of a king. The magical character of the stones also appears to have had a cosmological connection for the Persians.

In the great Assyro-Babylonian epic Ishtar's Journey to Hell, the precious crystals and gems worn by the Mother Goddess are sung about; among others is her girdle made of nephrite the "birthing girdle". At the fifth gate of the Underworld, the goddess had to take off these stones, called alan aladi, in order to pass through.

Another ancient Assyrian text gives an incantation for an ornament that should be set with seven gems and worn by kings as amulets. These gems and their effects were so highly thought of that they were even presented to the gods as amulet stones. The magic formula says:
"Shining, splendid stones; shining splendid stones; stones of joy and of luck glowing splendour for the flesh of the gods the Hulalini stone, the Sigurru stone, the Hulalu stone, the Sandu stone, the Uknu stone, the Dushu stone, the precious Elmeshu stone, perfected in celestial beauty. Laid on the King's shining breast as an ornament Azagsud, High Priest of Bel, make them shine, make them glow Protect this house from Evil."

The only stones mentioned in this spell that we can identify with some certainty are the Uknu, a lapis lazuli, and the Elmeshu, the most precious of the seven, the diamond.

These ancient oriental, magical-mythological interpretations of precious stones, crystals and gems continued to influence the cultures within the melting pot of Middle Eastern peoples – including the Jewish traditions in Palestine and, through them, on to Christianity.

Israel

> "... I will build you with stones of turquoise, your foundations
> with saphires. I will make your battlements of rubies, your gates
> of sparkling jewels, and all your walls of precious stones. All your
> sons will be taught by the Lord, and great will be your children's
> peace. In righteousness you will be established."
>
> Isaiah 54: 11-14

Throughout the entire Middle and Near East, kings, priests and other dignitaries adorned themselves with breastplates inlaid with precious gems.
Numerous burial finds from the Pharaonic period provide graphic evidence
of this. Of the highest cultic significance was the breast shield decorated
with twelve precious gems worn by the high priests of the Mosaic and post-
Mosaic periods, and for whom something like "gem oracles" existed. Before
the Babylonian Exile, this oracle served the Jews as a means of interpreting
God's will. In the Old Testament there is a detailed description of how the
breastplate should be made according to the will of Jehovah: "It is to be
square - a span long and a span wide - and folded double. Then mount
four rows of precious stones on it. In the first row there shall be a ruby, a
topaz and a beryl; in the second row a turquoise, a sapphire and an emerald; in the third row a jacinth, an agate and an amethyst; in the fourth row
a chrysolite, an onyx and a jasper. Mount them in gold filigree settings."
Exodus, 28, 16-20

The "sacred" number twelve of the stones - which, in this context, symbolised the twelve tribes of Israel - is also evident in the entire Mediterranean world: for the twelve signs of the zodiac as well as for the twelve
Olympian gods of Ancient Greece. The origins of this belief in twelve goes
back to Mesopotamia, and even the Egyptians had incorporated this number in their religion. The spiritual centre of Ancient Egypt was made up of a
priesthood, who also had the task of observing the stars and planets. In the
clear air, in which the moons of Jupiter could be seen with the naked eye,
this was an important task for a people, who lived mainly from agriculture.

The division of the calendar into twelve months also influenced their mythico-religious development: the number twelve was seen as an eternally repeating principle, willed by the gods themselves.

Although none have actually been discovered archaeologically in the Holy Land itself, precious gems are nonetheless often mentioned in the Old Testament. The conclusion is that they must have been imported from other countries and cultures. Judging by their names, jasper, beryl and lapis lazuli came from Mesopotamia, whilst carnelian, amethyst, hyacinth and turquoise, came from Egypt.

Another section in the Old Testament contains the description of "the Son of Man", who, on the day of his creation, was decorated with precious gems. "You were in Eden, the garden of God, every precious stone adorned you: ruby, topaz and emerald, chrysolite, onyx and jasper, sapphire, turquoise and beryl. Your settings and mountings were made of gold; on the day you were created they were prepared." Ezekiel 28; 13. The interesting thing is that the *New International Bible* used for the quote here uses different names for the precious stones than those in the earlier Bible translation. This rather leads one to deduce that the old terms for the stones must have been, for the most part, difficult to translate from the Greek or Latin.

The brilliant stones of "the Son of Man" have been interpreted as being the results of an ancient legend of the stars. The myth of the "fallen angels" (or precious stones) has also been connected with the signs of the zodiac. Here, we find the origins for later practises of assigning certain stars to certain precious gems. Indeed, it seems highly likely that the ancients knew about the precession of the equinoxes much earlier than is generally acknowledged. This is a process whereby the sunrise point of the spring equinox (and also the autumn equinoxe and solstices, of course) is gradually moving backwards through the twelve constellations of the zodiac in a huge 26,000+ year cycle (one degree of a zodiac sign about every 72 years). If the constellations of the zodiac were seen to be or to represent the gods (the stars being the stones etc.), then the Sun would have "visited" each constellation in turn over long periods of time, emphasising that particular god's status and the ever-shifting emphasis on different gods and the take-over of power from one god by another.

The Old Testament also gives us many other instances of the use of and the meaning of precious gems in ancient Israel. The prophet Ezekiel had a vision in which he saw behind the "foundations of the heavens" above the Earth, and "seven mountains made of precious stone". In his account, a throne appeared before him in the heavens, as if made of lapis lazuli. Similarly, the prophet Enoch spies a heaven made of crystal. Humans had learned the manufacture and use of jewellery and precious gems from the fallen angel, Azazel. More detailed mentions are also made in the Old Testament of the status of the gem-cutter and the goldsmith: "Then the Lord said to Moses, 'See I have chosen Bezalel son of Uri, the son of Hur, of the tribe of Judah, and I have filled him with the Spirit of God, with skill, ability and knowledge in all crafts – to make artistic designs for work in gold, silver and bronze, to cut and set stones..." Exodus 31; 1-5

If one regards the Old Testament as giving directions for the Jewish religious lifestyle, one can accept the fact that the wearing of precious stones was only allowed in connection with the divine, as any kind of profane use of this sacred material would have been rejected.

Ancient Greece and Rome

"If you could look at it from above, the true earth is like one of those balls made from twelve pieces of leather – variegated, and picked out in different colours... The same again with the mountains and rocks the earth has, which are correspondingly more beautiful in their smoothness, transparency and colour. The precious stones which are so highly prized here – cornelian, jasper, emerald, and so on – are fragments of these."

From Plato's Phaido

Precious gems were not always held in quite the same degree of esteem in Greece and Rome. It was not until the classical era of Hellenism that a wide range of stones was worked. Previously, much simpler stones, like steatite, (a type of soapstone) – for example– and some types of chalcedony had mainly been used.

The Persian Wars, which introduced the religious beliefs and spiritual customs of the Persians to the Greeks, were decisive in the development of the Greek art of working gems and for the new esteem in which gems were held. In this way, the Greeks also learned of the Persian ideas of the secret powers of precious stones, gems and crystals. This all then became part of the culture and literature of the Hellenist and late-classical era.

Finally, in ancient Rome, the old art of working gems experienced a highpoint, along with a great variety of types of stones being worked.

In the splendour of Imperial Rome, hard crystals such as diamond, ruby, sapphire, topaz, aquamarine, chrysolite, lapis lazuli as well as malachite and turquoise were particularly admired and were very popular. Various different types of chalcedony were also used, including among others, carnelian, jasper, agate, onyx and heliotrope – as well as amethyst and rock crystal.

The precious gems worked in Rome came mainly from the East. Arabia and Ethiopia provided amethyst, topaz, obsidian, and heliotrope; Crete supplied coral agate. Rock crystal came from Cyprus; emeralds and jasper from Asia Minor. However, the greatest proportion of precious stones came from Babylonia and from more distant countries, such as Persia and even India. In fact, during the Imperial Era, India supplied diamonds, rubies, sapphires, opals, lapis lazuli, tourmaline and beryl, among others to Rome. Even in antiquity, it was known that India was a huge source of such stones. This dates from around 120 BC, when Greek seafarers brought home precious stones along with spices from this far distant country. Roman literature refers to Indian precious stones as symbols of pomp and luxury.

However, a large part of the Roman demand for gems was met closer to home. Agate was found in the River Achates on Sicily, and amber came from the Ligurian coastline, (although it is still not clear whether this was the original source site, or merely a much-frequented trade centre for this commodity).

As in earlier cultures, the colour, brilliance and origin of the stones formed the basis for their identification and order in Rome. In addition to their important functions in decorative jewellery on clothing and the body – such as in the form of brooches, chains, rings and bangles – precious gems in antiquity also served as splendid decoration in architecture. In the construction of important temples and palaces – for example, in the Roman Palace of Jupiter for Psyche – the floors were adorned with them. During the Imperial Era, the Roman Capitol, which had previously been decorated only with foliage, was adorned with precious stones. The first Roman Emperor, Augustus (63 BC to AD 14), patron of the arts and a lover of precious gems, consecrated the largest rock crystal in the then known world on the Capitol. The crystal weighed more than 50 pounds (nearly 23 kg). The working of the stones in ancient Rome was carried out then in much the same manner as it is today. After the stone had been given the desired shape through cutting and polishing, it was often engraved, before being re-polished and then placed within a setting by a goldsmith.

The myths and legends about the secret powers and origins of precious gems had reached Greece via Asia. In turn, they also influenced ideas in ancient Rome. For example, there was a belief that chalcedony had been created through a "divine rain"; and even that haematite had come from the blood of Uranus, when he was wounded by Cronos. Agate had the reputation of helping pearl fishers; if it were thrown into the sea, it would be attracted by pearl oysters.

In order to waken the magical powers sleeping in gems, they had to be consecrated, with strict rules – celibacy among them – and instructions for care had to be observed. The stone was "given a soul" through magic formulas; it "talked" to the person who wore it and who saw it "breathe". However, the oracular power of the stone would fail if the wearer allowed it to fall on the ground. It is also recorded that it was forbidden to take off consecrated stones. Further, it was forbidden to pollute them – either through touching them or bringing them into contact with the dead.

The magical powers of precious stones also rendered them interesting to litho-therapy, about which the chapter on the healing powers of stones and crystals gives more information. This form of healing envisaged that the stones should be worn as amulets, or that they should be pulverised and mixed with salves and healing beverages. In the form of amulets, the stones themselves provided the required influence. However, as with the Gnostic "Abraxas gems", their influence could be heightened through an image carved into them or via a carved inscription. A special magical power was ascribed to each gem.

In antiquity, precious stones were connected with stars or planets, as they had been in Sumeria and Egypt. The light of the stars and the Sun were seen in their brilliance. In the Jewish *Talmud*, Abraham was given a precious stone by God, with which he could heal the sick. After Abraham's death, according to the story told by the Talmudist, Abbaji, God gave the stone to the Sun, which, in turn, increased its power.

Christianity and the New Testament

> "... before me was a throne in heaven with someone sitting on it. And the one who sat there had the appearance of jasper and carnelian. A rainbow, resembling an emerald, encircled the throne."
>
> Revelation, 4: 2-3

In contrast to the Old Testament, the New Testament only rarely mentions precious gems and pearls. Its overall teaching was that the pomp of this world was to be despised and only heavenly treasures should be praised and worshipped. However, in contrast, the New Testament records that when preaching the gospel, St. Paul did remind his companions that as well as the precious gems they should use only materials (figuratively speaking) that could withstand the fires at the Last Judgement.

St. John does not refrain from mentioning precious gems and crystals. In the Book of Revelation, the "New Jerusalem" is surrounded by a wall that gleams: "... [like] a jasper, clear as crystal. " This wall is built out of twelve layers of precious gems.

In just what manner these crystals penetrated the religious ideas of Christianity is demonstrated by the following description:

"The wall was made of jasper, and the city of pure gold, as pure as glass. The foundations of the city wall were decorated with every kind of precious stone. The first foundation was jasper, the second sapphire, the third chalcedony, the fourth emerald, the fifth Sardonyx, the sixth carnelian, the seventh chrysolite, the eighth beryl, the ninth topaz, the tenth chrysophase, the eleventh jacinth and the twelfth amethyst." Revelation 21: 18-21

Anthroposophists, who have spent much time unravelling the relationships between people and the mineral kingdom, perceive in the final book of the New Testament, the Revelation of St. John and the Apocalypse, a representation of the human sphere being penetrated by the mineral sphere. For them, the physical, sensory appearance of precious gems and crystals carries with it something that corresponds to the spiritual appearance.

In particular, the fourth chapter of Revelation describes God on his heavenly throne as compared with a jasper and carnelian, surrounded by an emerald rainbow. For the anthroposophist, this represents the symbolic representation of the identity of the physical appearance of precious gems and the spiritual appearance of God.

In spite of all the changes in specific meanings, each precious gem has never lost that symbolic value ascribed to it from time immemorial. During the era of early Christianity, the duality between the biblical challenge to reject earthly treasures, and the equally biblical acknowledgement of precious gems as a purified gift of God, favoured the adoption by the Christian Church of the symbolism of precious gems into its philosophy and worldview.

The Middle Ages

> "Every creature is burdened with the sin of the first man, especially the precious gems, which God has created, like the herbs and many other things, for the use of man. The powers of the precious gems are damaged through the handling and use of them by impure, sinful humans."
>
> Konrad von Megenberg, 1309-1374

In the Middle Ages, earlier ideas and concepts from antiquity about the nature of precious stones and gems were, for the most part, taken further and described in detailed treatises - for example, by the mystic, Hildegard von Bingen, by Albertus Magnus and by Agrippa von Nettesheim.

Far from employing "empirical science", which might have cast doubt on the old descriptions of the classical authors, - for example, the notion that a diamond could be "split asunder by the blood of a ram" - the authors would speculate ever anew about how precious gems could have been created: "Every gem has fire and moisture in it. The Devil shows terror, hatred and contempt towards the precious gems. This is because they remind him that their brilliance already existed before he had been toppled from that splendid position God had bestowed on him, and also because some gems are created in the very fire, in which he has to suffer the torments of his punishment." Hildegard von Bingen

In the Middle Ages, religious ideas were still strongly influencing the sciences - so that this attempt at explaining the creation of precious gems is not really surprising. However, the mystic, Hildegard von Bingen (c. 1100-1179), was already making an attempt at interpreting the origins of crystals from more than just a religious angle.

To her, certain natural phenomena appeared to be the basis for the creation of precious stones, gems and crystals. In her work, entitled *Physika*, she writes the following: "Precious gems are created in the East and wherever the sun shines hottest. The mountains in such regions retain heat like fire from the Sun's energy, and the rivers there are thus always hot, so that

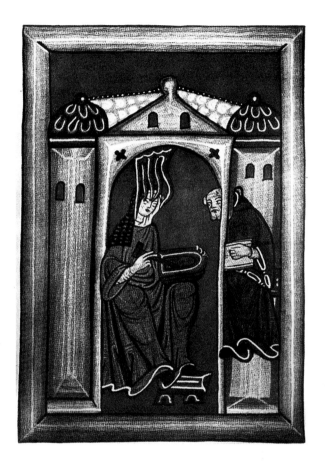

The abbess, Hildegard von Bingen (c.1100-1179) writes down her attempts to explain the creation of precious gems in her work, Physika, as depicted here in a miniature from the codex Scivias.

occasionally a flood breaks out from these rivers, and the flood rises up to those mountains. The water touches the mountains, which are also glowing with heat from the Sun's energy, and where the water and fire meet, foam is thrown up, as one can observe with molten iron or melting-hot stone... Then the 'foam' sticks and hardens over three or four days and turns to stone. Then, when the flood of the waters recedes, so that they return to their bed, this 'mud', which has remained adhering in different places in the mountains, dries out, depending on the times of day and the temperature. Depending on the temperature at the time of day, the 'mud' obtains its colour and energy and hardens into precious gems. When a further flood of the rivers occurs, they pick up numerous such stones and crystals and carry them away to other lands, where they are finally found by humans."

The frequent mention of precious gems and crystals in the *Bible* influenced the medieval way of describing and interpreting gems and crystals and affected both poetry and the general accepted wisdom of the times.

Many authors in the Middle Ages were occupied with allegorical interpretation of the twelve precious gems of St John's account of the Apocalypse, with more attention being paid to their colour than to their physical reality.

The Venerable Bede, an English religious scholar of the late seventh–early eighth century, interpreted the specific verse of the Apocalypse and remarked that each of the twelve precious gems was a symbol for the foundations of the "New Jerusalem". However, he did ascribe certain qualities to individual gems as follows:

"Jasper refers to the greening of faith... In chalcedony we see the flame of inner love..... in beryl the perfect actions of the prophets. Topaz reveals their glowing performances... This means the individual gems are assigned to the individual foundations, and although all are perfect, through which the city of our Lord is decorated on its holy mountain, but they glow with the light of spiritual mercy."

In eleventh century Europe, there was a widening of knowledge about precious stones, crystals and gems. The so-called "Lapidaries", books about crystals and stones, were compiled on the basis of ancient sources. In these, the first consideration was not only the allegorical interpretation of the names of the precious gems, but also their magical powers. Their colours

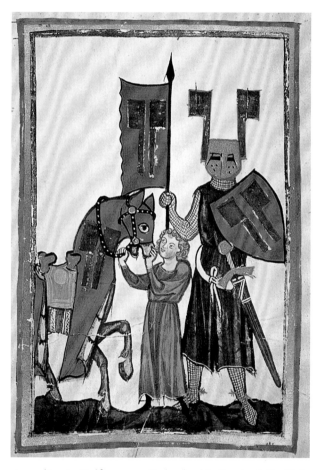

According to Wolfram von Eschenbach's Parzival, the Holy Grail was supposed to have consisted of a single, huge precious stone. This likeness of the poet is a miniature from the Manessian manuscript (1300–1340).

played an extremely important role in all of this. For example, red crystals were connected with blood. Thus, the carnelian was thought to be able to staunch bleeding and almandine was believed to fortify the circulation. Similarly, the green emerald was thought to heal the eyes and improve vision.

Furthermore, magical powers were not only ascribed to the particularly outstanding crystals, but also even to less conspicuous ones, such as for example, antimonite. People in the Middle Ages believed seriously and piously in what they perceived to be the wondrous powers of gems.

The legacy of the associated beliefs from the late-classical period was mixed with pagan and Christian culture, such that wherever additional support was required for the imagined effects of certain stones, the same formula was always quoted: that God had given the precious gems their wonderful powers, which should not be doubted. Hildegard von Bingen wrote about this as follows: "And just as God won back a better fate for Adam, so He also prevented the beauty and power of the precious gems from being lost forever; moreover, He wished them to remain on Earth as an honour and a blessing and as a means of healing."

The scholar Dominican Albertus Magnus (1193-1280) argued in a similar way to Hildegard. He did not doubt the wonderful powers of precious gems and he was certain that they could have the power of healing stomach ulcers and other complaints. However, Albertus also tried to explain this academically and was at pains to substantiate the traditions of antiquity with his own experiences and observations. He maintains that he had seen a carbuncle that glowed in the dark, and that a sapphire healed a person suffering from an eye disease.

The imaginary, so-called "carbuncle stone" had a central and commanding role among gemstones throughout the entire Middle Ages, as it was considered to have within it the concentrated powers of all the other noble gems. It was ascribed with having the ability to glow in the dark, and it was said that it grew at the base of the horn of the fabled unicorn. Thus, the "carbuncle" became a symbol of divine light on earth. This image was fed mainly by medieval literature. In the world of the Middle Ages, it was also represented by rubies, the red spinel or a correspondingly vivid red garnet.

Throughout this era, the belief in the multi-facetted miraculous powers of gems never faltered. The theological interpretations also influenced medieval poetry and the field of high courtly love. For example, in Gottfried von Strassburg's *Tristan und Isolde* (c. 1210), the bed in the grotto of courtly love consists of rock crystal, a symbol for purity.

Again, in Wolfram von Eschenbach's *Parzival* (c. 1210), there is a further impressive example for the significance of precious gems in medieval literature. The Holy Grail, which plays a central role in this epic, is said to have consisted of a single, huge gemstone – unambiguous in intention, with its several references to the "carbuncle stone". The connection with the divine seems especially clear here, as the Grail is a holy vessel and is connected with the Christian Eucharist. However, Celtic pagan elements are also associated with its function. Therefore, finally, the Grail has clear magical funtions: it bestows eternal youth; it is too heavy to be lifted by the uninitiated; it serves as an inexhaustible provider of food; is invisible to pagans. In addition, it sometimes displays a holy message on its surface, which disappears spontaneously as soon as it has been read.

Yet, the Grail itself is not the only precious stone mentioned in Parzival, for the bed of the Grail King, Amfortas, is described as being set with 58 precious gems, all of which possess magical powers.

Examples indicating the significance of precious gems in medieval literature could be cited almost ad infinitum. Their significance was eminent and always connected with magical ideas, which were to be retained for centuries. Indeed, the magical properties associated with precious gems were also favoured by medieval alchemy. This "science" represented a transition from the mythical worldview of antiquity to present-day material scientific research. It saw the nature of the Earth and humans as a microcosm, a reflection in miniature of the universe, which was the macrocosm. Alchemy pursued the refinement of distillation as a process for the purification of natural substances – but its ultimate goal was to obtain the most noble and precious of all stones, the "stone of the wise" or so-called "Philosopher's Stone".

Naturally, throughout the Middle Ages, precious stones played an extremely important part in the search for the Philosopher's Stone, the lapis philosophorum or lapis occultus. Both the aforementioned "carbuncle" and the Holy Grail had already been associated alchemically with this stone, so conferring on it a form of divine status. In a parallel context, the Philosopher's Stone was also sometimes referred to as the "elixir of life". This was thought not to be something found in Nature, but rather something that had to be obtained through various alchemical processes. Such procedures had to follow a sequence, at the beginning of which was the secret prima material, and the final result of which was the perfectum magisterium, or the completed masterpiece. The "pure vessel", which was needed for creating this item – and also for the much-attempted creation of gold out of base matter – consisted merely of rock crystal. Alchemy also gave rise to many notable and diverse activities, such as the use of spheres and balls made of so-called "white crystal" that served as a means of fortune telling and the use of antimonite to separate gold and silver.

The preparation and knowledge of The Philosopher's Stone were said to be the secret of only a circle of initiates. This gave rise to the alchemists' frequent reference to lapis noster or "our stone" However, whilst this was an artificial product in reality, the alchemists emphasised that it in itself demonstrated their belief that there was no distinguishable difference between art and nature. In the fourteenth century, Hortulanus explained it as follows: "In the same way as the World was created, Thus is Our Stone manufactured."

In their search for the legendary lapis occultus, the alchemists tried to remove all impurities from the then known precious gems, and thus to "purify" matter. The instructions for these experiments were often expressed in secret illustrations, which only an initiate knew how to interpret. One interesting idea stemming from this work of the alchemists was that precious stones grew just like plants.

Preparation of healing substances was another important field of study and activity within alchemy, and the lapis occultus was ascribed healing and rejuvenating powers. Unfortunately, it was never discovered.

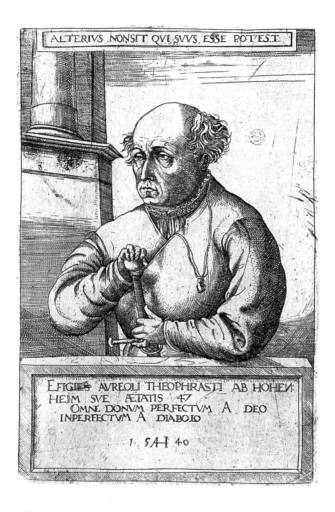

ALTERIVS NONSIT QVI SVVS, ESSE POTEST.

EFIGIES AVREOLI THEOPHRASTI AB HOHEN:
HEIM SVE ÆTATIS 47
OMNE DONVM PERFECTVM A DEO
INPERFECTVM A DIABOLO

1. 5A+ 40

*The physician and philosopher, Paracelsus, real name
Theophrastus, lived from 1493 to 1541. Among the extensive
investigations carried out by Paracelsus, the healing power of
precious gems played a central role.*

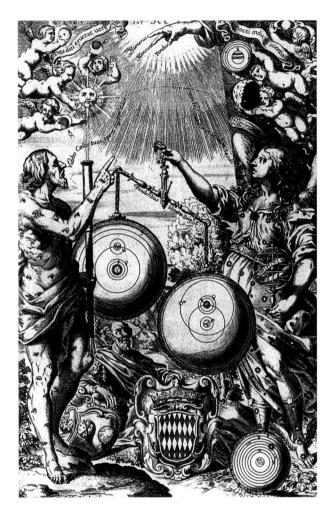

The various solar systems as envisaged and proposed by Copernicus, Tycho Brahe and Ptolemy are represented in the above illustration.

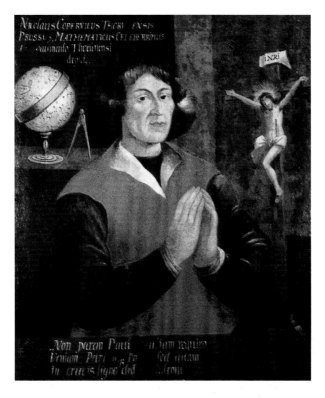

Nicholas Copernicus (1473-1543) worked out the heliocentric view of the world by describing the annual movement of the Earth around the Sun, and explained the daily revolution of the heavens with the fixed stars as the rotation of the Earth around its own axis. Nevertheless, this did not mean that metaphysical thought was in any way abandoned.

The Modern Age

> "The stone was an opal,
> Which provided a play of a hundred beautiful colours,
> And had the secret power
> Of making whoever carried it with faith and trust
> Appear pleasant in the eyes of God and humans."
>
> Lessing, Nathan the Wise ("The Ring Parable")

By the sixteenth century, the philosophy of humanism had evolved a completely new concept of the world and nature – and, correspondingly, ideas about precious stones and gems. This concept was also linked with an altered view of antiquity.

Thus, while mainly late-classical sources had been used for the investigation of precious gems during the Middle Ages, the new thinking resulted in references being made to the works of authors like Pliny and his description of natural history (in the first century), which appeared to stem from an even earlier time.

People such as Erasmus of Rotterdam, Ulrich von Hutten and Philip Melanchthon are among the best-known humanists, but there were many among them, especially physicians, who were especially interested in the healing powers of gems and crystals.

For the first time, historically speaking, humanists did not baulk at the notion of criticism when examining the work of the classical and late-classical authors. Their study of classical sources, however, was one of the most important foundations in the development of a new concept of the sciences. Specifically, in the context of gems and crystals, Georgius Agricola (1494-1555) is considered to be the founder of what was then the new study now called mineralogy. He set aside the fields of religion, magic, astrology and philosophy and studied the actual appearance and physical nature of individual minerals, crystals and gemstones.

Paracelsus (Theophrastus Bombastus von Hohenheim, 1493-1541), a German physician and Renaissance philosopher, and a contemporary of

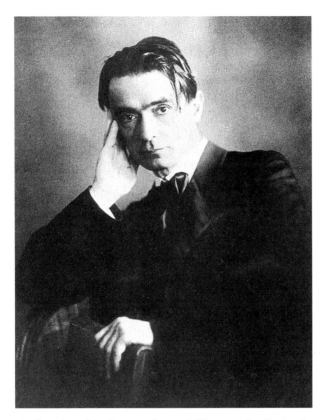

The founder of anthroposophy, Rudolf Steiner (1861-1925).
His teaching gave crystals and gemstones a special status.

Agricola, is best known as a multi-disciplined natural scientist and the founder of the newer science of healing substances. The art of healing with precious gems and crystals played an important part within his research. He perceived human beings and minerals as part of a world seen as a whole and as a work ordered by God.

The Baroque era of the seventeenth century, leading into the eighteenth century, brought about a renewal of scientific thought in which its points of departure were empirical research and a pantheistic philosophy.

Naturally, in such a climate, mineralogy was also affected by this philosophy and, consequently, humanism had a decisive influence on this whole period.

One of its most conspicuous characteristics was the perceived paradox or contrast between elaborate artwork (including the creation of jewellery) on the one hand, and the contempt for all worldly things, on the other hand. Based mainly upon religious perceptions, the Earth was seen as a "vale of suffering", a mere antechamber to the real life, the 'beyond'. The concept of vanitas mundi, the "vanity of the world", in which all is mortal, stems from this era, which was also characterised by important scientific discoveries and a rise of the bourgeoisie after the Thirty Years War (1618-1648) had torn Europe apart.

While the Paracelsian renewal of the Neo-Platonic legacy had led to attempts to create a magical-alchemical total view of God and the world, the burgeoning sciences of astronomy and mathematics were influencing a whole new body of thought in considering the natural world. This is typified by the likes of Copernicus and, later, Kepler, who revealed a whole new view of the world when they formulated the heliocentric basis of the solar system. However, this did not lead to any immediate anti-metaphysical overview. Rather, it was seen as simply liberating oneself from the scholastic dogma and freeing the mind from the old bonds, chains or shackles of theology.

Curious as it now seems, the efforts to represent the world as an orderly whole also led to a renewed interest in astrology and numerology, as is evidenced within literature of that period. Belief in the magical powers of precious stones, etc., had been central in the medieval art of healing and in the field of the spiritual-cum-sacral. Now, the very same minerals were not only the objects of mystical nature and the worship of God, but also the subject of scientific observation. However, metaphysical thought had not been pushed aside by any means. Instead, such ideas simply survived all the historical processes and continued to exist alongside the new concepts and approaches, right to the present day.

The teachings of anthroposophy, developed by Rudolf Steiner in the twentieth century, form a link between humans and the spiritual principle of the universe. Here, humans are meant to connect with and allocate a unique position for crystals and precious stones.

This concept corresponds with Steiner's ideas of the "secret sciences" and the principles of higher worlds. He describes gems as follows:
"...sensory organs of higher spiritual beings ... through which these beings, which have no physical bodies, obtain the possibility of looking into the earthly-physical happening ... This occult fact was known to the priest-kings of pre-history, and to many of the great initiates."

Throughout time, we have always revered gems, crystals and precious stones and elevated them materially and spiritually into objects of respectful contemplation. They have always been ranked according to different degrees of value, though this order of importance has changed throughout history and been rather different from one culture to another. An indication of this, as we have already seen, is how the "carbuncle" occupied the highest position in medieval Europe as a legendary stone for its marvellous powers.

Finally, the present-day definition of a gemstone was created in the eighteenth century, when Urban Friedrich Benedict Brückmann wrote:

"Precious gems is the term given to those stones which, because of their transparency, hardness, stability, smoothness or by their ability to take on a beautiful gleam through grinding, rarity, and because of their beautiful colours, excel above others... and the more such characteristics are possessed by a stone, the more perfect it is considered to be."

Nowadays, in all cultures and societies, the above can be seen to apply perfectly to the diamond as being generally regarded as the finest of all gems, especially for a stone cut with facets and polished to assist its brilliance. However, the emerald enjoys a unique reverence, which happens to correspond with the healing and magical effects that are ascribed to it.

Precious gems are worn by many people, not only as items of jewellery – or as a form of capital investment – but also because of the mysterious powers that have always been attributed to them – those of protection, healing and as bringers of luck.

Gemstones and the Zodiac

From very early times - several thousand years BC, in fact - connections were being made between precious gems and heavenly bodies, in both Mesopotamia and Ancient Egypt. It was assumed that the energies of the seven (then) known planets could also be found in corresponding precious stones. Thus, the gems became thought of as being "stars on Earth", each having a close correspondence with its associated "star" and also being assigned to the corresponding constellation of the zodiac.

However, many (and often rather different) opinions existed about which gems were assigned to which sign of the zodiac. Generally, it can be said that all these interpretations have a common basis - the relationship between the macrocosm of the Universe and the microcosm of humans and the natural world, for which one wanted to create a close and intimate connection.

Nowadays, with historical and cultural hindsight, we suppose that it was most probably the Sumerians who originally laid the foundations for the astrological principles that describe the Sun's course through the twelve signs of the zodiac - and which influences the Earth and human behaviour. The symbolism and the effects, which were ascribed to the planets and constellations, then led to certain gems being incorporated in this system. The Sumerians also saw a connection between the constellations and developments in nature and the cycle of the seasons. The constellations were used as signs for sowing and harvesting and as symbols for the dry and rainy seasons.

Other cultures, too, have used these same cycles in their respective mythologies and cultural connections, with the constellations being transferred into symbols of the respective culture. Stellar constellations were also connected with precious gems in the advanced civilisations of Asia Minor.

The reverence shown towards "sacred" or "holy" gems in the traditions of Mesopotamia and Egypt also influenced the cultures of the Greeks and Romans. The ancient "lapidaries" - books about gems and crystals - of

Rome provide many interpretations and much wisdom about gems and crystals. However, classical interpretations are numerous and vary a great deal. As a result, no single or unified interpretation can be identified. Nevertheless, one thing they all have in common is the belief in a "sympathetic" correspondence – so that certain characteristics match up with certain organic (and inorganic) substances, including the heavenly bodies.

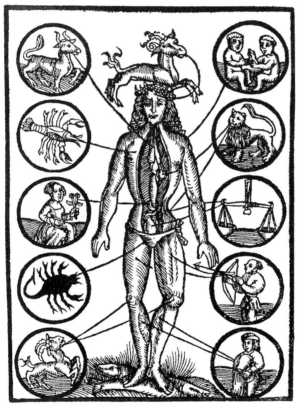

A manikin, that shows points on the body for "bleeding" (or cupping) a sick person, together with information on the astrologically advantageous times during which to carry out the procedure.

Putting it all together, this meant that crucial elements of the worldview were seen in relation to each other, while still taking into consideration basic characteristic features – including the four "temperaments". The four elements also played an important role, as they were assigned to the above-mentioned forms of expression – even if in a sometimes somewhat far-fetched manner – in order to depict the desired and unified worldview. This, in turn, created the concepts of "sympathy" and "antipathy".

The microcosm and the macrocosm were among the leading elements of the imagination in the classical, philosophical worldview. Completely in line with this was the thinking of astronomer and geographer Ptolemy (who lived from the year 87 to165 and whose ideas were based upon ideas from antiquity and were then developed further in the Middle Ages), in which the Earth was seen as the centre of the World; the Earth was believed to be surrounded by a number of spheres, one within the other, and each of which influenced the one below it. According to Ptolemaic teaching, "the influences of God's almighty powers" penetrated all these spheres, all the way down to we humans on Earth.

It was assumed that gems and crystals were formed via the influence of fixed stars and were thus able to transfer or transmit waves and energies from the macrocosm to the microcosm. This meant that precious gems were ascribed a sacred significance, in which secret powers also played a part. Agrippa von Nettesheim (1486-1535), whose work *De Occulta Philosophia* was strongly influenced by classical sources – and was for centuries of the foremost significance for astrology and the mantic arts – made connections between the twelve gems of the Apocalypse (in the Book of Revelation) and the twelve signs of the zodiac:

Aquarius – rock crystal	Leo – jasper
Virgo – emerald	Pisces – sapphire
Aries – sardonyx	Libra – beryl
Taurus – carnelian	Scorpio – amethyst
Gemini – topaz	Sagittarius – zircon
Cancer – chalcedony	Capricorn – chryosprase

The main planetary influences are the basis for these so-called "correspondences". In the case of gemstones, it was their emitted light spectrum that was the decisive and most important property.

Anthroposophy, a discipline that has emerged in modern times, sees a connection between the spiritual and the everyday natural world. For example, anthroposophy occupies a position that validates links between gems and the signs of the zodiac. Looked at another way, the months of the year and established seasonal festivals can only be interpreted if the appropriate relationships are seen not merely from the activity itself, but also from the spiritual background (or its origin and empirical purpose), which was believed to have been the case in the "ancient mysteries".

Steiner, the main founder of anthroposophy, believed it and staged it as follows "...the common and shared basis for precious gems and crystals, humans and the starry heavens is the spiritual effectiveness of the hierarchy of the Cherubim (spirits of harmony), whose creative impulses, differentiated through lower spirit beings, appear as the material cosmos". In fact, according to Steiner, they differentiate the twelve main forms of the animal and plant kingdoms in what he termed a "creating" manner.

However, there is an assumption here that the problems encountered again and again when trying to assign precious stones, gems, etc. to the signs of the zodiac, all originate from the fact that there was no single "twelve" precious gems. Rather, there were only seven – in accordance with the seven formerly known (or named) planets and their associated "spiritual effect" – which now can be seen to modify those of the conventional twelve signs of the zodiac.

Numerous traditions exist as to which gem is assigned to which sign of the zodiac. The calendar months have shifted through time with respect to the constellations of the zodiac. This phenomenon is known as the precession of the equinoxes. Thus, one may find working lists of gems belonging to the months, as well as gems belonging to the signs of the zodiac, Some of them differ significantly from each other, as they are based on different original sources.

Because of the equinox precession, henceforth we will deal here only with the gems connected with the modern twelve signs of the zodiac, as they no longer correspond to our present-day calendar months.

Nevertheless, the astrological tradition also makes connections between individual planets and certain gems. These gemstones are supposed to be lucky for those people with the corresponding planets occupying a favourable placement in their birth horoscopes.

Most modern lists of gems and corresponding zodiacal signs only provide the reader with a table, without any more detailed explanation. However, set out below is a brief overview, with a description of the links between the zodiacal signs and their associated gemstones. Furthermore, closely linked with this is the analogy of the planets, their corresponding zodiacal signs and certain colours. The symbolic values of these colours are also the basis for an evaluation of the identified gems, not least because of the actual wavelengths and electro-magnetic (spectral) frequencies that lie behind the light scattering properties of gems and what we perceive as their colours.

As only seven planets were known in ancient times (at least, in Europe), the spectrum was identified with only seven colours. In turn, these were assigned on the basis of them assuming the existence of four elemental basic colours – red, yellow, green and blue. Added to these were the precious metals gold and silver (as colours,) along with black, (although, in essence, it is not a colour at all). In this way, the following planetary colour correspondences were designated:

Mars – red	Saturn – black
Sun – gold	Jupiter – blue
Venus – green	Moon – silver
Mercury – yellow	

The "pure" colours were assigned, accordingly, to the "fire signs", as follows: red to Aries, blue to Sagittarius, yellow to Leo.

The astrological tradition assigned one planet to each sign of the zodiac, and which was thus thought to influences human fate. According to the sources we have, and which do indeed differ somewhat from each other, one still finds nevertheless the following, recurring associations between the signs of the zodiac, colours, planets and gemstones:

Aquarius 21 January – 19 February
Colour: blue/green
Planet: Uranus
Gems: aquamarine, turquoise, labradorite, falcon's eye, amazonite

Pisces 20 February – 20 March
Colour: violet, blue, opal shades
Planet: Neptune
Gems: amethyst, blue Sapphire, blue moonstone, opal, kunzite

Aries 21 March – 20 April
Colour: red, reddish
Planet: Mars
Gems: ruby, carnelian, fire opal, red Garnet, Jasper

Taurus 21 April – 20 May
Colour: light red, brownish, orange
Planet: Venus
Gems: salmon pink sapphire, zircon, orange carnelian, light-coloured sapphires, light-coloured agate, rose quartz, chrysocolla

Gemini 21 May – 21 June
Colour: yellow, orange, greenish
Planet: Mercury
Gems: yellow sapphire, yellow and green beryl, topaz, peridot, citrine, amber, tiger's eye

Cancer 22 June – 22 July
Colour: silver, white, green
Planet: Moon
Gems: emerald, opal, moonstone, chrysoprase, chalcedony, nephrite, pearl

Leo 23 July – 23 August
Colour: white, yellow, gold, reddish
Planet: Sun
Gems: diamond, chrysoberyl, white zircon, gold-coloured citrine, pink topaz, rock crystal

Virgo 24 August – 23 September
Colour: yellow/greenish
Planet: Mercury
Gems: yellow diamond, yellow sapphire, tiger's eye, emerald, jasper (various colours), and citrine

Libra 24 September – 23 October
Colour: blue/reddish
Planet: Venus
Gems: indigolith, aquamarine, salmon-pink coral, blue topaz, star sapphire, jasper, kunzite

Scorpio 24 October – 22 November
Colour: black/red
Planet: Pluto
Gems: opal (black precious), red spinel, rubellite, sard and sardonyx, red corals, haematite, malachite

Sagittarius 23 November – 21 December
Colour: blue
Planet: Jupiter
Gems: lapis lazuli, dark-blue spinel, blue zircon, blue apatite, chalcedony, sodalite

Capricorn 22 December – 20 January
Colour: green/black
Planet: Saturn
Gems: green tourmaline, malachite, chrysoprase, onyx, black coral, pearl, moss agate

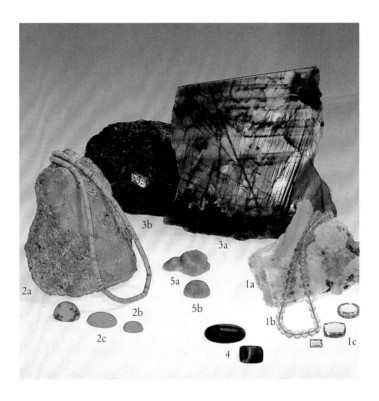

AQUARIUS

1 Aquamarine
1a Crystal in matrix
   (Pakistan)
1b Necklace of beads, transparent
1c Three facetted gems, (Brazil)
2 Turquoise
2a Large rough stone (Arizona)
2b Necklace of cylindrical
   Turquoise beads (Arizona)
2c Three cabochons (USA/Iran)

3 Labradorite
3a Sawn and polished slab
   (Madagascar)
3b Rough stone
4 Falcon's Eye, two cabochons
   (South Africa)
5 Amazonite
5a Group of crystals (Colorado)
5b Cabochon (Brazil)

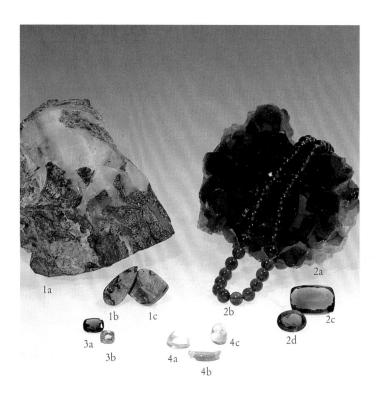

PISCES

1 Opal

1a Opal in matrix
   (Australia)

1b Polished Opal with matrix
   (Australia)

1c Polished Opal with matrix
   (Australia)

2   Amethyst

2a Group of crystals (Brazil)

2b Necklace of beads (manufactured
   in Idar-Oberstein, Germany)

2d Facetted gem (Brazil)

3   Sapphire, blue

3a Facetted gem, (Sri Lanka)

3b Facetted gem, (Sri Lanka)

4   Moonstone, blue

4a Cabochon (India)

4b Cabochon (India)

4c Cabochon (India)

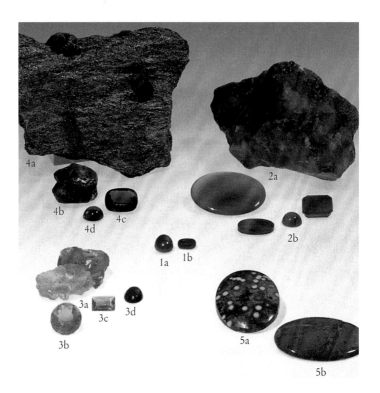

ARIES

1 Ruby
1a Cabochon (India)
1b Facetted stone
   (Myanmar/Burma)
2 Carnelian
2a Rough stone (Oregon, USA)
2b Four different cabochons (Braz.)
3 Fire Opal
3a Two different coloured rough
   stones (Mexico)
3b Large facetted stone (Mexico)

3c Facetted stone (Mexico)
3d Cabochon (Mexico)
4 Garnet, red
4a Garnet crystals in rock
   (Alaska)
4b Rough stone (Madagascar)
4c Facetted stone (Madagascar)
4d Cabochon (India)
5 Jasper
5a Spotted Jasper (USA)
5b Red Jasper (India)

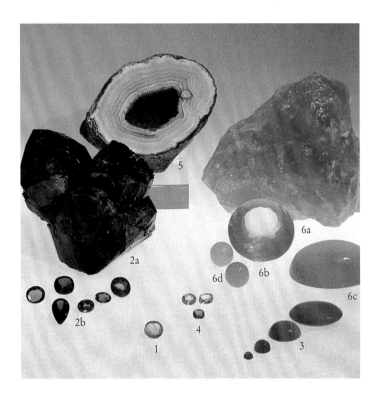

TAURUS

1 Sapphire, pink, red-orange
   facetted stone (Sri Lanka)
2 Zircon
2a Group of crystals (Norway)
2b Six facetted stones
   (Cambodia/Sri Lanka)
3 Carnelian
   different size cabochons
   (India/Brazil)

4 Sapphires, different colours
5 Agate, lightly polished stone
   (Fischbachtal, Germany)
6 Rose Quartz
6a Rough stone (Brazil)
6b Facetted stone (Brazil)
6c Cabochon (Madagascar)
6d Two spheres (Brazil)

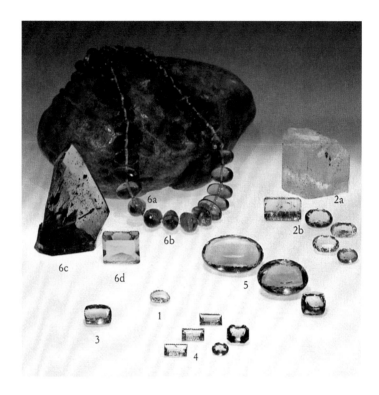

GEMINI

1 Sapphire, yellow
  facetted stone (Sri Lanka)

2 Beryl, yellow, colourless, green

2a piece of broken crystal (Brazil)

2b Five facetted stones (Brazil)

3 Topaz
  facetted Precious Topaz (Brazil)

4 Peridot
  five facetted stones
    (USA/Myanmar/Burma)

5 Citrine
  three facetted stones (Brazil)

6 Amber

6a Rough piece (Poland)

6b Necklace
    (Dominican Republic)

6c Lightly polished rough piece
    with fossil inclusions
    (Dominican Republic)

6d Facetted Amber (Dominican
    Republic)

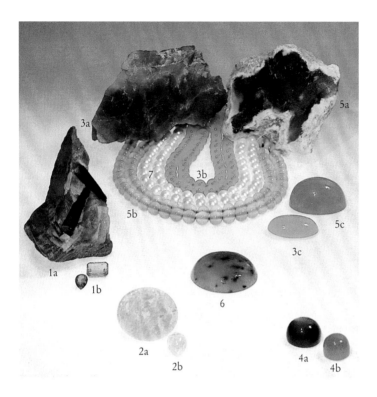

CANCER

1   Emerald
1a Emerald in matrix (Columbia)
1b Two facetted stones (Columbia)
2   Opal
2a Cabochon (Australia)
2b Cabochon (Australia)
3   Chrysoprase
3a Rough stone (Poland)
3b Necklace of beads
3c Cabochon (Australia)

4   Moonstone
4a Greyish cabochon (India)
4b Salmon-coloured cabochon
       (India)
5   Chalcedony
5a Rough stone (Brazil)
5b Necklace of beads
5c Cabochon
6   Nephrite cabochon (China)
7   Pearls necklace (South Seas)

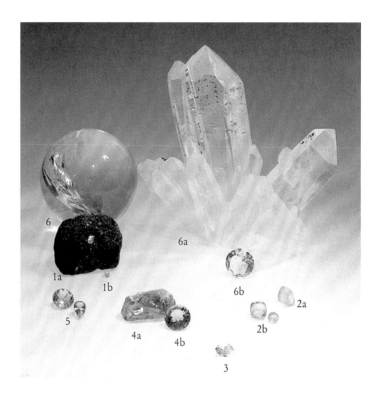

LEO

1 Diamond
1a Crystal in matrix (South Africa)
1b Diamond, facetted
   with special diamond cut
2 Chrysoberyl
2a Rough stone (Minas Gerais,
   Brazil)
2b Facetted stone   (Minas Gerais,
   Brazil) and a cabochon
3 Zircon, white
   facetted stone (Thailand)

4 Citrine, gold-coloured
4a Rough, unworked stone (Brazil)
4b Facetted stone (Brazil)
5 Topaz, pink
   two facetted stones (Brazil)
6 Rock Crystal
6a Group of crystals (Diamantina,
   Brazil)
6b Facetted stone (Brazil)

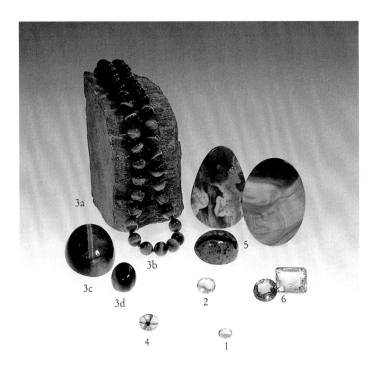

VIRGO

1 Diamond, yellow
  facetted stone (South Africa)
2 Sapphire, yellow
  facetted stone (Sri Lanka)
3 Tiger's Eye
3a Rough stone (South Africa)
3b Necklace of beads
3c Large cabochon
3d Cabochon

4 Emerald (Trapiche)
  (Columbia)
5 Jasper
  three different coloured
  cabochons (USA)
6 Citrine
  two facetted stones (Brazil)

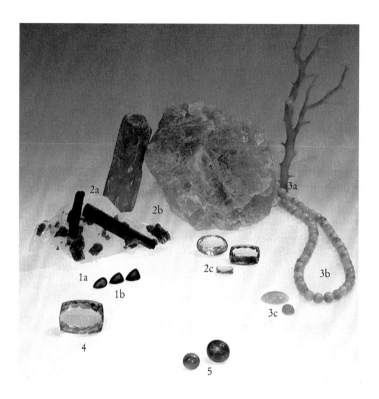

LIBRA

1 Indigolith (Tourmaline, blue)
1a Crystals on Quartz (Minas
   Gerais, Brazil)
1b Three facetted stones (Minas
   Gerais, Brazil)
2 Aquamarine
2a Rolled crystal from river gravel
   (Brazil)
2b Crystal in Quartz (Brazil)

2c Three different size facetted
   stones of various qualities
   (Brazil)
3 Corals, salmon coloured
3a Coral tree (Japan)
3b Bead necklace
3c Two cabochons
4 Topaz, blue; large facetted stone
   (Brazil)
5 Star Sapphire
   Two cabochons (Sri Lanka)

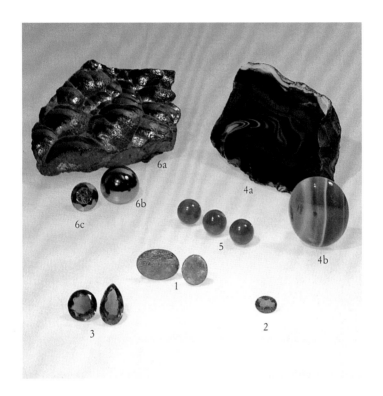

SCORPIO

1 Opal, black Precious Opal
  two cabochons (Australia)
2 Spinel, red
  facetted stone (Myanmar)
3 Rubellite (Tourmaline, red)
  two facetted stones
  (Madagascar)
4 Onyx
4a Lightly polished piece
  (Brazil)

4b Cabochon (Brazil)
5 Coral, red
  three balls (Mediterranean)
6 Haematite
6a Rough stone, lightly polished
  (Cumberland, Britain)
6b Cabochon (Brazil)
6c Facetted stone (Brazil)

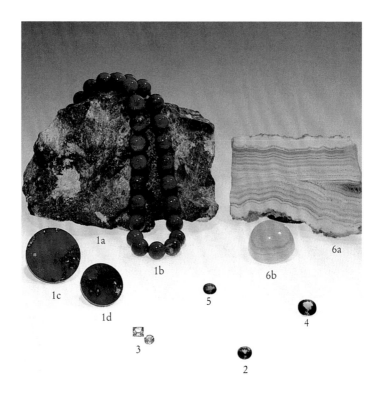

SAGITTARIUS

1 Lapis lazuli
1a Rough stone (Afghanistan)
1b Bead necklace (manufactured
    in Idar-Oberstein, Germany)
1c round plaque with Pyrite
    inclusions (Afghanistan)
1d Small round plaque
    (Afghanistan)
2 Spinel, dark blue
    facetted stone (Sri Lanka)

3 Zircon, blue
    two facetted stones
4 Tanzanite
    facetted stone (Tanzania)
5 Apatite, blue
    facetted stone
6 Chalcedony
6a Lightly polished rough stone
    (Brazil)
6b Cabochon (Brazil)

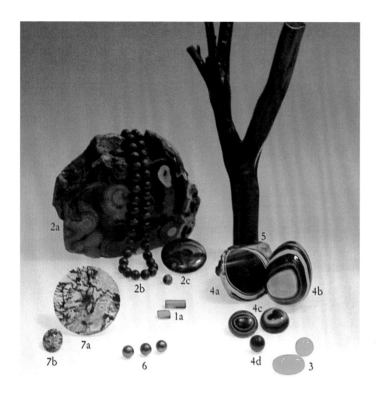

CAPRICORN

1 Tourmaline, green
1a Two facetted stones (Brazil)
2 Malachite
2a Lightly polished rough stone
    (Zaire)
2b Bead necklace (from Idar-
    Oberstein, Germany)
2c Two cabochons (Zaire)
3 Chrysoprase
    two cabochons (Australia)
4 Onyx

4a Lightly polished rough piece
4b Egg (made of Onyx)
4c Two cabochons
4d Sphere, drilled
5 Black Coral, lightly polished
    black branch (Dom. Republ.)
6 Black pearls, three pearls
    (South Seas)
7 Moss Agate
7a Large slab, polished (India)
7b Cabochon (Brazil)

Amulets and Talismans

In his *Westöstlichen Diwan*, in the 'Book of the Singer', Goethe chose sardonyx as a talisman, along with agate and its colour zones – black onyx in the background, white between and red carnelian above:

"Talisman of Carnelian,/lends luck and health to those who believe; if it's on an Onyx base, kiss it with a consecrated mouth! All evil is driven away thereby, Protects thee and protects the place."

From the very earliest times we seem to have tried to create for ourselves "magical armour" in order to achieve protection from danger and from the natural world. Since those times, people have also made considerable effort to determine exactly which individual stone or mineral might be lucky for the individual. Not surprisingly, the choice of which to wear as talismans was often made with the help of the zodiacal circle.

As a result, astrology was closely bound up with the fear that our forbears had about their unknown fate and possible dangers. By extension, it has always been of great significance for those striving for protection and actually trying to 'direct' their own fate, if at all possible. However, especially in ancient times, "reading the stars" in this way was not just seen as a way to predict both the future and one's fate; it also served as a way in which to interpret the world and the cosmos in its entirety.

Ever since the flourishing of the advanced civilisation of the Ancient Egyptians, it has been customary to produce talismans and amulets "at the right moment" – namely, when the respective planetary aspects were deemed to be favourable.

One example of these "magical glyptics" comes from the sixteenth century, where the manufacture of amulets and talismans played an important role. At the time, the Arab scholar Hunain ibn Ishaq wrote the following:

"The Bloodstone is assigned to Mars. It is a red stone. Whoever takes this stone on a Tuesday, while the Moon is in opposition to Mars in the sign of Aries or Scorpio, may manufacture a stone for a ring out of it, and engrave an image of Mars on it. It should depict a naked man, at whose right side is an image of Venus, whose hair is knotted behind... Then the stone must be set in an iron ring, as iron and copper are assigned to Mars... No-one may withstand the wearer of this ring; neither a robber nor a wild animal may approach him, and people will revere and love him."

In Goethe's time (1749-1842), a distinction was made between an amulet and a talisman. While the talisman often consisted of a gemstone on which a name or a short verse was engraved, an amulet was a gem or crystal without any engraving and that was placed inside a small bag, along with a separate, written invocation. Soldiers, in particular, were recommended to carry such amulets during times of war.

Amulets were supposed to ward off the "evil eye", i. e. to overcome and vanquish demonic powers and the violence of enemies. They were also supposed especially to protect the wearer from poisons and dangerous animals. Talismans, on the other hand, were not intended to ward off threats or dangers, but to attract love, luck, good health, power and wealth.

During much of the period covered by stories in the Old Testament, the Babylonians already had amulets to ease pregnancy and labour in childbirth, and to protect children. In turn, this influenced the Hebrews and precious gems assumed a new importance for them. It was often the practice to wear pieces of jewellery directly or in a small bag next to the skin – in the form of rings, necklaces and bracelets – as an equivalent to the protective or magical character of an amulet.

Equipping amulets and talismans with signs and engraved verses is a special art. To learn it requires a thorough and intensive study of numerology, runes, symbolism, the Kabbalah and astrology.

Letters of the alphabet, syllables, words, sentences, numbers and signs are all elements of magic used in this art form – with the Hebrew alphabet and the teaching of the Kabbalah playing an especially important role.

The Nordic runes were also important as symbols used for empowerment in their own traditions, and in Indian culture the mantric syllable Om was, and still is, of great significance in this context.

The decisive factor in deciding the material from which a talisman or amulet was made was often the choice of whichever gems could be linked with certain planets and thus, with the zodiacal sign, of the wearer.

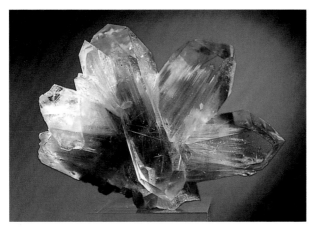

Rutile star within quartz crystals, Brazil

A well-known verse from a lucky amulet of Phoenician origins, says: "Adonis, hear my words and bless my work, as you are the ruler of the Earth and the Heavens, the true ruler, who will return with the Age of Bliss."

A Chaldean/Aramaic verse expresses it as follows: "My Lord will not lay any illnesses upon me."

A vast variety of amulets existed in the ancient Middle East. In evaluating grave goods, it is clear that this tradition continued through the Egyptian, Hellenic and Roman civilisations and on into the period after the great migrations, arriving finally in Europe around the sixteenth and seventeenth centuries. Here, the talismanic tradition and medicinal healing were seen as being complementary, and treatments often incorporated the use of precious gems and crystals.

In medieval Europe, the instructions for the creation of amulets or talismans from precious gems or crystals frequently included one to lay the gem in a gold or silver vessel that was to then be filled with white or red wine, and allowed to stand in moonlight for three nights. Then, the wine, which was regarded as being charged with the energy of the precious gem, was to be drunk and the stone was to be used for making an amulet.

Important astrological considerations when making such a talisman or an amulet were to incorporate information from the personal horoscope of the prospective wearer. These included such elements as the Ascendant sign, the planets occupying the first house, and the positions of the Sun and the Moon. In doubtful cases or when there was insufficient information, a pendulum was often used and its swing consulted in order to determine the choice of the particular precious gems to be used.

These days, the characteristics ascribed to amulets or talismans tend more to be linked with our hopes for the present and the future. This is rather different from the way in which earlier amulets or talismans were regarded, i.e. when they were based on a magico-religious ideas and beliefs. Nevertheless, personalised objects are still seen as the bringers of luck and continue to have significance for many people, even in today's so-called "civilised", modern world. After all, it is clearly a deep rooted human desire to wish to add that extra "something" to any favouring of individual good fortune, success and security – even if the modern wearer is not now always so certain about the real effects of these secret little charms.

Crystal and Gemstone Healing

"A precious gem hung
from the neck of
our father, Abraham,
and every sick person
who saw him
immediately became well again."

Talmud

Because there are many titles specialising in nothing but crystal therapy, only a basic outline of the general principles and healing effects of precious stones, crystals and other minerals gems can be dealt with here. The specific healing powers ascribed to them are summarised in the alphabetical listing (pages 88 – 155) in more detail.

The early, initial fascination with crystals and gems was based almost entirely upon their physical beauty – their colours, almost perfect transparency and light-reflecting qualities.

In the early stages of most developing cultures, an array of practical instructions evolved as to how and in what manner to use precious stones and crystals as treatments for certain illnesses and ailments. For example, malachite powder was believed to help with pains in the limbs and to cleanse the eyes.

Gradually, these highly pragmatic fragments of advice turned into fuller, complicated systems and theories. Thus, it became no longer just a matter of prescribing malachite powder. In addition, there were stipulations as to the time of day at which to take the powder and who should administer it. Shamans and medicine men, for example, used the crystals and gems in cult-based ceremonies and rituals, such as worship of the Moon. Healing thus shifted into the realm of suggestion and auto-suggestion.

In India, in particular, precious gems have always been employed as a medium of healing. In Ayurvedic philosophy (ayurveda, an ancient Hindu word meaning something like "the science of life") there are numerous references to such therapies in which patients took the gems in a pulverised form. Naturally, only a small, affluent and privileged group were able to afford this, as the gems could not be used again and were very expensive to purchase in the first place.

Gems were also often worn externally for their healing effect. This involved placing them on the diseased part of the body, or by stroking and massaging the relevant area of the body with a gemstone. Naturally, these methods were far less costly and, accordingly, applicable over a much broader range of the population. Healing salves and tinctures were also prepared from grinding crystals and gems, with ground pearls, sapphires, malachite and stibnite/antimonite being particularly in demand for such preparations.

Colours too played an important role in crystal and gem therapy. According to the ancient principle similia similibus curantur (meaning something along the lines of "healing like with like"), the colour of the gem in question was decisive for the relevant healing method. Thus, red, the colour of blood was important for treating diseases of the blood and its circulation, and for the healing of bleeding wounds. A good example of this occurs in the *Hortus Sanitatis* (1486) of Johannes of Kuba, where the following instruction can be found for staunching a nosebleed:

"Ematites (haematite), bloodstone:... this stone is cold and dry in nature. This stone, taken in the hand, when there is a nosebleed, will staunch bleeding from the nose. This stone, pulverised and mixed with Shepherd's Purse juice and applied in the nostrils, will remove the bleeding there from."

The knowledge of crystal and gem therapy had come to Europe via Arabic culture. It was usually assumed that the more precious a gem, the more effective its healing powers would be. Even critical scholars, who warned about superstition and deception, still did not doubt these basic healing powers. From Zoroaster to Theophrastus, from Pliny to Albertus Magnus, and from Agrippa von Nettesheim right through to the nineteenth century,

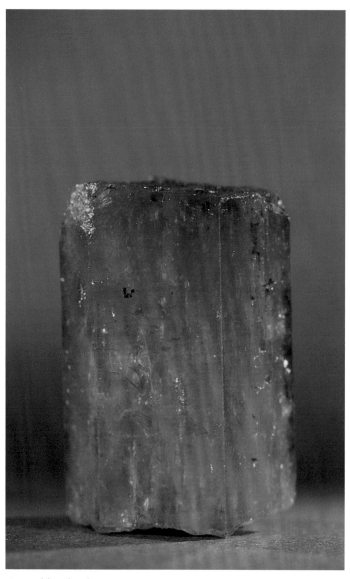

Emerald, Columbia

the healing powers of gems and crystals was recognised, accepted and much described. Even down the centuries, the actual instructions for their use was only ever partially modified.

In an instruction manual dated 1696, we find the following quote:

"For the preparation of a gem: the precious gems/such as ruby/emerald/hyacinth [zircon] and garnets are first burned in a melting pot. Then dowsed in rose water and dried. Then ground up into powder first on a grinding stone then in a mortar, together with rose borage and similar heart-fortifying waters. Then ground down even more finely/Then dried."

The beauty and perfection of gems - at least, in comparison with any items made by human hand - led people to believe in the divine, healing powers of gemstones and, in turn, come to connect them with conceptions and notions such as power, strength and protection. Inevitably, this led to their use in the healing arts.

According to ancient Indian traditions, the human body possesses seven important power centres, the so-called "chakras", through which cosmic energy influences the body. This actually "nourishes" the person - or rather the chakras themselves, which then influence the whole body. If the body does not obtain sufficient energy this way, the result is ill health. Each of the seven chakras has its own characteristics and influence; but all are interconnected.

This radiation, in turn, is divided up into "coloured rays", which also appear in the rainbow, and various gems have been assigned to these colours. This was how the distribution of gems to certain organs of the human body, which, in turn, were assigned to the relevant chakras, evolved.

According to this ancient Indian view, the necessary cosmic colour energy can be transferred to a patient with the help of the relevant gemstone or crystal, so that natural energy equilibrium is restored within the body. Gems and crystals play an important role as healing agents in Ayurvedic practice, which includes detailed descriptions about which gems are to be used for which ailments and illnesses. The colours identified in cosmic radiation energy are those of the spectrum - violet, indigo, blue, green, yellow, orange and red. For example, red, being considered the colour of fire - that which radiates heat - meant that red energy sources were meant to warm the body.

Based on the traditional Indian chakras, W. A. Tiller of Stanford University, California, in 1975 assigned certain allegedly healing gems to different organs of the body. For example, to the head he assigned diamond, emerald, sapphire, ruby and moonstone. Further, sapphire was assigned to the bridge of the nose; diamond was connected with the throat and neck; precious topaz and ruby to the heart; red coral to the abdomen (the base chakra).

Nowadays, the art of crystal healing is once again very much in vogue - both as therapy and in research. Interestingly, this may well be due in part to the fact that the chemical composition, crystallographic configuration, atomic structure and electromagnetic properties of minerals and their trace elements are now known - paralleling many of the characteristics that were already guessed at and exploited long, long ago.

The Earth's Genesis
Geological Timescales

Any interest in minerals and their finest forms – crystals and gemstones – requires at least some basic background knowledge of their origins. Any study of rocks and minerals is inherently connected with their genesis and the Earth's geological development into the way we know it today.

Further, in order to explain and understand the history of the Earth involves trying to grasp the idea of time spans of many millions of years. Our own limited time span shows just how impossible it really is to get to grips with such a concept. In many ways, this is well demonstrated by the image created by the words of Hendrik van Loon in *The Story of Mankind*: "Way up north in the land of Svithjod, there is a rock. It is 160 kilometres tall and 160 kilometres wide. Every one thousand years, a small bird arrives on this rock, in order to sharpen its beak. When the whole rock has been ground away in this manner, only a single day of eternity will have passed by." As even a mere 1000 years is virtually unimaginable to us, even the above image can still only serve as an approximation of the true aeons of the time during which the Earth evolved.

Modern scientific opinions and assumptions are that some 4.6 billion years ago, a celestial body began to form out of cosmic dust through the actions of primal physical energies. This body heated up to many thousands of degrees and became liquid.

During this stage, there was a "sorting" process of elements and compounds that was a result of and in keeping with their relative densities. Heavy metals, such as iron and nickel, sank into the depths and formed the nucleus of the Earth. Lighter components, such as silicon compounds, became concentrated at higher levels and continued to build up the approximately 2,700 km-thick layers called the mantle. From the Earth's mantle, through magmatic processes, the very top layer of about 8-40 km separated out as the Earth's crust. In turn, from the various types of rock of which it is made, all of the known minerals were formed.

For the last fifteen years, the gneiss rocks from western Greenland have been dated as being about 3.8 billion years old, and were considered to be the oldest rocks on Earth.

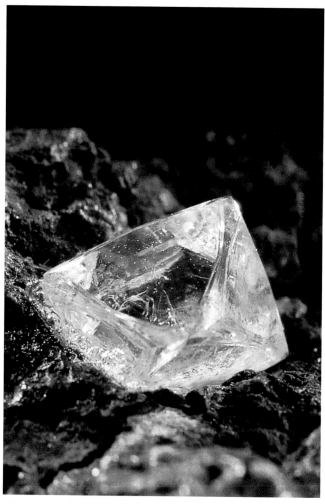

Diamond within kimberlite rock, South Africa

More recently, thanks to newly developed dating methods involving the measurement of inherent radioactivity; scientists can now determine the age of different kinds of rocks with considerably more accuracy. As a result, dates of 4.2 billion years have been cited in published scientific journals, etc., including such minerals as eclogite in South African kimberlite.

In another case, grains of zircon have been dated at about 4.55 billion years old in younger Australian rocks. Meanwhile, other investigations - of Moon rocks and meteorite material - have resulted in information about the "missing" period that constitutes the postulated first 0.4 million years of the Earth's existence.

Minerals are substances that have arisen through natural geological processes. They are characterised by having a unified composition and are almost always of a solid consistency. They are nearly all made up of one or several basic unique "building blocks" of matter - the chemical elements themselves. Every element, in turn, has its own atomic structure made up of neutrons, protons and electrons.

Minerals can consist of an individual element as well as of combinations of elements. For example, diamond is probably one of the best known of all minerals (as well as being renowned as a beautiful gemstone). It consists solely of the element carbon (C), and so is no different - chemically - from any other form of carbon, be it graphite or particles in soot: it is the arrangement of the carbon atoms themselves that creates the form (called an allotrope) that we call diamond.

Taking another compound example, the precious gems known to us as ruby and sapphire belong to the corundum group, which consists of the elements aluminium (Al) and oxygen (O), bound together in a ratio of 2:3. All therefore have the chemical formula Al_2O_3, but can appear in various physical forms - including the hard crystalline form we know as gem-stones.

Because of their origins and differing geological conditions and factors - such as heat, pressure or the available material - crystals are formed which may be as large as a metre or more. Equally, they can just as easily be only a few millimetres in size.

Crystals are three-dimensional, solid bodies with a regular internal arrangement of atoms. In most cases, they exist in a strictly geometrical configuration called a crystal lattice. In turn, it is this type and structure of the crystal lattice that determines the crystal surfaces, which are the outer surface limits of the mineral. In fact, it is the crystal lattices that endow minerals with their own particular physical and chemical characteristics, which we will consider in more detail below (page 79 - 85).

The energies that help to create the colours, shapes and types of these wonders of nature are processes not easy for the layman to understand. Nevertheless, they are of considerable interest, as the magic of a crystal or gem – which can touch us deeply on several levels of feeling – cannot be explained by science alone. It is a beauty that will always be experienced in a very personal way, yet remains a mystery.

Mineralogy

What we know as mineralogy, along with its associated science of crystallography, has had a long evolution throughout human civilisation and culture. This is well worth looking at, albeit briefly, in order to provide a valuable context for what follows.

History

Records and accounts of minerals exist from the times of the Ancient Greeks and Romans. Aristoteles (384-322 BC) describes both minerals and metals in his work *Meteorologica*. The Roman author, Pliny the Elder (23-79 AD), in his *Natural History* consisting of 37 volumes, dedicated a total of four volumes to minerals.

Only much later, towards the end of the Middle Ages, were the first comprehensive scientific works written, laying the foundation for "mineralogy", as it came to be known.

The term "mineral" itself is almost certainly derived from the Latin minare, meaning of obtaining of a substance "from a mine or quarry" – demonstrating the close historical connection between the words and activities of "mining" and "miner".

Modern mineralogy belongs to that field of study termed the geosciences and has always been the basis for the search and exploitation of raw materials. It also has the task of bringing order to, and an explanation of, the natural material that surrounds us on all sides.

An interest in minerals has always been a vital theme for humankind – as raw materials, building materials, for making objects and for jewellery and decorative items. However, our interest here is limited to just a small section of the Earth's minerals – namely the precious stones, gems and crystals used for jewellery and for healing.

Precious stones and gems can be defined roughly as those minerals, which, because of their special characteristics, have been highly prized by humans. Among these characteristics are their hardness, purity and rarity, display of colours, brilliance and conspicuous luminosity.

Nearly all gemstones only reveal and display their full beauty after they have been expertly polished, and modern techniques enable a gem to shine with its full, brilliant fire.

The term "semi-precious" stone used to be employed in the gem trade for less expensive gems, i.e. those suitable for making less expensive types of jewellery. However, modern terminology is restricted to the use of just "decorative stones" or "precious stones", where the decorative stones can also include bio-organics like pearls, amber or coral.

The following categories are used in listing the characteristics of a precious stone or gem:

- Name
- Group
- Colour
- Hardness
- Specific gravity
- Crystal system
- Crystal shape
- Chemical composition
- Origins and occurrence (deposits)

For more detailed explanations, see pages 88 - 156.

Names

The names of many minerals and their crystals originated from the ancient Greek, Latin, Arabic, Indian and even (occasionally) European languages. The commercial world of the gem trade has also introduced further imaginative names in order to promote sales, creating a situation whereby a mineral or precious stone is sold under two, or even several, names. This has now been corrected and unified, with terminology rules for crystals, precious stones and gems having been established nationally and internationally.

Some common examples for the origins of names include malachite, which is derived from the Greek word mallochitis lithos, "mallow stone". Diamond is from the Greek adamos, "the invincible"; tourmaline is from the Singhalese words meaning, "red precious gems"; ruby comes from the Latin rubeus, "red".

Groups

Mineral groups are what we call minerals with the same, or similar, crystal structure, but with variable chemical compositions. Additionally, trace elements can also cause variations in degrees and shades of colour.

The corundum group provides a good example of this type of occurrence. So-called "common" corundum is a mineral containing a mixture of the elements aluminium and oxygen in the ratio $2:3$ and so, as aluminium oxide, all have the chemical formula of Al_2O_3. They are grey in appearance, being basically colourless but ranging to a light bluish shade. Their great hardness means that they are used almost exclusively as grinding materials. If forms of corundum occur with very slight traces or inclusions of the metallic elements chromium or iron and titanium, they acquire a colouring and become what we call rubies or sapphires, with their red or blue colouring, respectively. In other words, it is only the inclusion and effect of these trace elements which causes the characteristic colouration.

The quartz group is another example, where coarse-crystal quartzes include rock crystal, smoky quartz, amethyst, citrine and rose quartz. Quartz varieties with inclusions are aventurine quartz, sapphire quartz, prase, tiger's eye and falcon's eye. Finally, there are the fine-crystal quartz aggregates such as chalcedony, chrysoprase, heliotrope, carnelian, agate, jasper and fossilised (petrified) wood.

Colour

Gems and crystals come in different colours and the colour often determines their worth. For example, a corundum that is only faintly red is not yet a ruby. It acquires that name only when it has an intense and characteristic red colouration (see earlier).

What we call light – white light – is actually composed of a series of electromagnetic wavelengths, which form the visible spectrum (red, orange, yellow, green, blue, indigo and violet). A ray of light passing through a crystal may be partially or totally absorbed by the crystal and it is these absorbed wavelengths that are observed as being "missing" from the emergent spectrum – so that, in combination, all wavelengths that are not absorbed create the perceived colour of the gem or crystal. If all wavelengths pass through the gem, then it appears to us as being white or colourless. Exactly which wavelengths are absorbed is determined by the mineral's content of metallic elements such as chromium, iron, cobalt, copper, manganese, nickel and vanadium. Often even the tiniest trace amounts of such inclusions of "foreign" substances are enough to give any crystal a different colour.

The way that a rough gemstone is cut and then highly polished, along with the shape and facets connected with this process, make its colouring all the more conspicuous and provide the characteristic "sparkle".

In the case of non-transparent or semi-opaque minerals – such as lapis lazuli, turquoise, etc., – the colour is determined by the same sort of absorption and reflection, but only on the gem's surface.

Hardness

This is the term used to characterise the resistance that a mineral offers against external mechanical pressure. The Viennese mineralogist Friedrich Mohs (1773-1839) chose ten minerals of varying, comparative hardness and assigned to them a succession of numbers from 1-10 as a measure of increasing hardness – the Mohs Scale. On the scale, diamond has a hardness of 10 and talc, as just about the softest of minerals, is ascribed a hardness of 1. Every mineral assigned to the scale has the property of being able to mark physically – to "scratch" – any that are lower in the scale.

All minerals have their own characteristic hardness. Thus, this is a physical feature that can be used to identify any mineral in question. Minerals with a hardness of more than 7 are best suited as jewellery, as they would otherwise be too soft for daily use – but even the finest dust contains quartz particles with a hardness of 7, which can damage softer types of crystal.

Specific gravity

The specific gravity (or relative density) of minerals is also a characteristic feature that aids categorisation and identification. Generally speaking, it indicates how much heavier a body is than the same volume of water at 4 degrees Celsius. It is expressed in units of weight per volume - usually as grams per cubic centimetre (g/cm^3).

Specific gravity is of great importance in the search for gems and rare or precious metals, as many can often only be distinguished from the naturally surrounding rock or ores by their greater density. Separation or extraction from rocks in which they occur or are found can involve a range of processes. However, some minerals accumulate through natural, physical processes and can then be found in natural locations, such as deposits or layers or rock veins. This is exploited, for example, when panning for gold. This process involves the swirling in water of gold-bearing sand in a flat pan until the lighter sand particles are washed out, leaving behind the heavier gold particles in the bottom of the pan. It was the main method adopted by the old-time gold prospectors, but is still in use in many parts of the world.

Crystal shape

In mineralogy - and more specifically in crystallography - crystal shapes are categorised as being one of seven basic configurations, each of which is derived from its basic, symmetrical structure. These are as follows:

- cubic
- tetragonal
- hexagonal
- trigonal
- [ortho]rhombic
- monoclinic
- triclinic

This division is helpful for a visual determination of minerals.

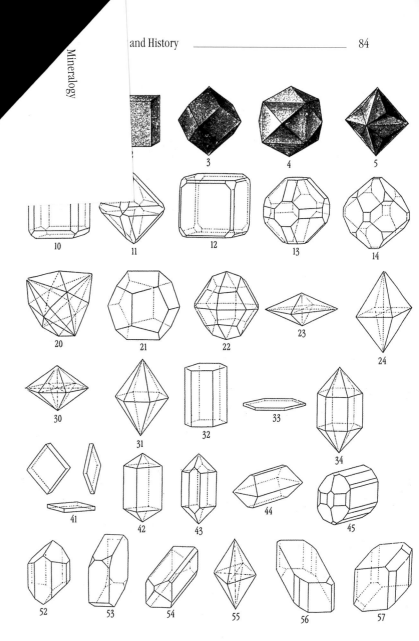

Crystal shapes and crystal systems
1-22: cubic; 23-29: tetragonal; 30-35: hexagonal;

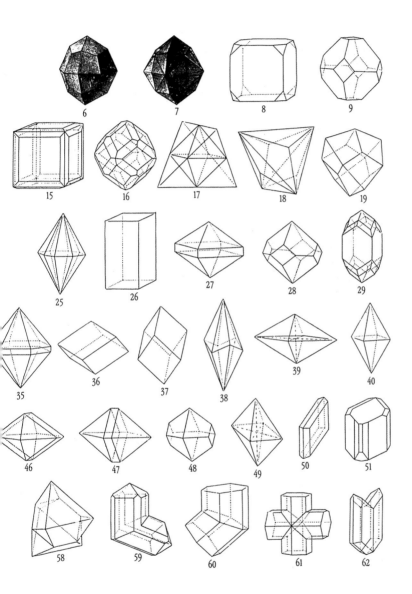

36-41: trigonal; 42-48: [ortho]rhombic; 49-54: monoclinic; 55-57: triclinic; 58-62 special shapes.

Chemical composition

Every mineral has a specific chemical formula, according to its basic elementary composition and indicates the relative proportions of the mineral's basic molecule. However, any trace elements, which are usually the source and cause of colour variations, are usually omitted from the basic chemical formula.

Origin, formation and natural deposits

Minerals can be formed by a wide variety of geological processes and stages – crystallising from solutions, by condensation of gases, from molten rock and lava, or even via the transformation of extant minerals. The starting points are always crystal nuclei, on which further elements or molecules are deposited and grow as long as the necessary conditions for crystal formation are present. We need not, however, continue to occupy ourselves here with the complicated chemical and physical processes which lead to the formation of or transformation of the minerals. In essence, there are three areas in which mineral formation takes place.

Igneous rocks – minerals originating from molten rock, from gases or from solutions in locations of magma-based formations

Metamorphic rocks – mineral formations, formed from other exiting minerals by pressure and/or temperature changes below the melting point of the other minerals.

Sedimentary rocks – minerals that arise in stratified environments or areas of formation.

Other enrichments, which have arisen through the concentration of certain minerals, are known as deposits; these may be either primary or secondary deposits.

With primary deposits, minerals are found in their unaltered state, preserved within the original rock formations.

In secondary deposits, minerals have been transported from the place of their origin by a process of erosion and re-deposited elsewhere as sediment.

Throughout this process, nature can appear to be "selective" during the transportation of eroded material, so that less dense minerals (those with a lower specific gravity) become separated from those with a higher specific gravity.

The concentrations of heavier minerals transported and deposited in this way - called alluvial deposits - are popular sites for gem hunters. If they are lucky, for example, diamonds may be found in either a primary or a secondary deposit.

Crystals and Gems A-Z

AGATE

It is alleged that a river called Achates, where the first agate was found, is the source of its name. Whether a real river or simply mythological, it was first described by the Greek philosopher Theophrastos (372-287 BC). The Arabs then brought large quantities of the crystal to Europe and it is their desert-originated culture and desert-like environments that gave rise to the idea that an agate held in the mouth helped to alleviate thirst. This ascribed property was then taken up in Europe and can be found in the medieval lapidaries.

Indian agates were especially famed, particularly for their allegedly beautiful picture-like markings, in which it was believed that animals and landscapes could be seen and identified. Wide-ranging healing powers were ascribed to agate and were even noted by Hildegard von Bingen (1098-1179) and Konrad von Megenberg (c. 1309-1374).

Green agate is supposed to help with curing certain eye complaints. Touching the precious stone was also believed to alleviate pain – and even lead to complete healing, if used constantly for treatment. It was also said to have a helpful effect on fevers, epilepsy and infertility. In modern crystal healing and therapy, agate is increasingly employed for easing headaches, lifting depression and treating skin diseases.

Magical powers are also ascribed to agate. Women are supposed to fall in love with men wearing the precious stone. Agate is alleged to bestow greater awareness, particularly on those born under the sign of Taurus, especially in their dealings with other people. It is supposed to help the wearer develop the ability to distinguish between "true and false friends".

Healing properties: helps with headaches, skin diseases and (especially) with feverish infections.

Astrology: Taurus; bestows greater sensibility. Capricorn (moss agate); strengthens willpower.

Name: Agate

Group: Quartz

Colour: various colours, with stripes and markings of reddish- brown and grey-blue shades; often artificially dyed (black, green, blue, etc.)

Mohs scale hardness: 7

Specific gravity: 2.6 (plus or minus 0.05)

Crystal system: trigonal

Crystal shape: crypto-crystalline aggregate

Chemical structure: SiO_2 silicon dioxide

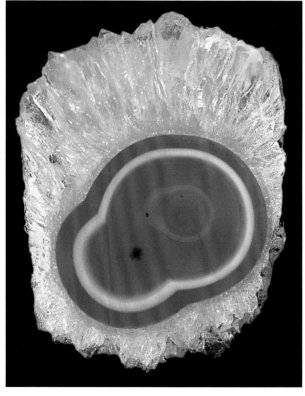

Agate with quartz, Brazil.

Natural formations: hollow spaces in volcanic rock
Important deposits: Brazil; Mexico; Uruguay; Germany (Idar-Oberstein); Indian sub-continent; USA.

ALMANDINE; see GARNET

AMAZONITE

The name of this crystal derives from some rather confused ideas at the time as to the name of the great river of South America. The explorer Alexander von Humboldt described in his travel records how he found some green crystalline material, known by the name "Amazon stones" among the native people of the Rio Grande. These crystals, which were very popular there and highly prized, were fashioned by the local people into a cylindrical shape, drilled through lengthwise, and worn around the neck as an amulet against snake bites and illnesses. They were often decorated with figures and inscriptions.

However, the original source of the crystals was not along the Rio Grande. According to what the Native Americans told Humboldt, they actually came from the "land of women without men, where the women live alone". Humboldt therefore linked this with the River Amazon in South America, where another early explorer, Francisco de Orellana, had battled with a tribe of Tapuyas, whose women fought alongside the men, as was the custom among the entire tribe. As a result, Orellana derived the name Amazonas from the Greek myths and legends of ancient Amazons, the warrior women of Asia and Africa that had been described by the Ancient Greek historians Herodotus and Diodorus – a circuitous route indeed.

Healing properties: for pains in the solar plexus area and for heart complaints.

Astrology: Aquarius; strengthens vitality.

Name: Amazonite
Group: feldspar group
Colour: green; bluish-green
Mohs scale hardness: 6
Specific gravity: 2.56 – 2.58
Crystal system: triclinic
Crystal shape: prismatic
Chemical structure: $K[AlSi_3O_8]$ potassium aluminium silicate
Natural formations: volcanic rocks and pegmatites (coarse-grained igneous rocks)
Important deposits: USA (Colorado); Madagascar; Namibia; Russia; Brazil.

AMBER

The Greeks gave amber the name elektron, possibly derived from the Phoenician word for sun, and so meaning something like "golden like the sun".

The Greeks also knew that amber could become statically charged through rubbing. The philosopher Theophrastus described this electro-static characteristic of this crystal in his lapidary, and the word "electricity" is derived from elektron.

These qualities of amber were interpreted in healing in such a way to indicate that it possessed astringent qualities. Arab doctors thus used amber for staunching nosebleeds. Pliny mentioned amber as an aid in preventing insanity and also recommended wearing it in the form of amulets to protect the wearer from a painful throat.

As a component of incense (amber in German is Bernstein and in Low German Brennstein, "burning stone"), it was also used against epilepsy and for driving away "bad spirits", as Konrad von Megenberg recorded in the Middle Ages. Amber was also believed to protect the wearer from asthma and rheumatism, and to strengthen the heart.

For those under the sign of Gemini, amber is like a "Sun", helping to enhance intuitive aptitude and the facility to recognise "true friends".

Healing properties: helps with asthma and rheumatism; strengthens the heart muscle.

Astrology: Gemini; the "sun stone", which boosts self-assurance and optimism.

Name: amber

Group: none

Colour: light yellow to brown, reddish, white, blue, greenish

Mohs scale hardness: 2-2.5

Specific gravity: 1.08 (plus or minus 0.02)

Crystal system: amorphous; no crystal lattice structure

Crystal shape: usually a clump or lump

Chemical structure: approx. $C_{10}H_{16}O$; mixture of different wood resins

Natural formations: amber is a fossilised resin formed mainly during the Tertiary Age and hardened in a sedimentary situation. Pieces often contain insects that were trapped in the sticky wood resin at the time and thus preserved for millennia

Major deposits: Russia; Baltic Sea coast; Dominican Republic

AMETHYST

"An amethyst is this stone;
I, Bacchus, am a drinker.
Either it will teach me sobriety,
Or it will lead me to drink."

Ancient Greek saying

All cultures appear to have ascribed great significance to the amethyst. In India, it was dedicated to the Buddha and monks in the monasteries of Tibet meditated with malas ("rosaries") of amethyst. In Arabia, it was venerated as a protective gem, often placed under the pillow to prevent nightmares.

The Greek word amethyein, which means approximately "not drunken", derives from certain characteristics assigned to it in classical times. The amethyst, the colour of which is rather similar to the stain left by red wine, was meant to protect from drunkenness – hence the custom, in antiquity, to drink wine from amethyst goblets. The classical name of the amethyst as the "Bacchus stone" was derived from the Roman version of an ancient Greek myth, according to which, the goddess Artemis (Diana) turned a nymph who was loved by Dionysos (Bacchus) into an amethyst.

In the Middle Ages, when the amethyst was worn by bishops and cardinals, it entered the medicine lore of the period. Hildegard von Bingen, for example, recommended it for improving the skin and even as protection against snakebite. Konrad von Megenberg believed that amethyst drove away "bad thoughts" and also stimulated the thought processes.

Not surprisingly, the idea that amethyst could heal alcoholism also lived on and in modern crystal therapy is used as an aid to boost powers of concentration and determination. It also has a calming effect on the heart and nerves and helps with sleeplessness and migraines, when stroked across the temples.

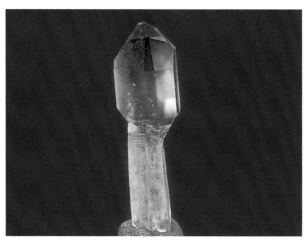

Amethyst (sceptre crystal)

In astrology, the amethyst is assigned to Pisces and is supposed to enhance the intuitive faculties of the wearer, as well as forming a "link to the cosmos". It is also alleged to enhance openness towards others as well as encouraging one's intellectual faculties.

Healing properties: induces a calming effect on the heart and nerves; improves the ability to concentrate; eases migraines and sleeplessness.

Astrology: Pisces; supports intuitive aptitudes and mental, spiritual and intellectual faculties.

Name: Amethyst
Group: quartz group
Colour: pale to deep violet
Mohs scale hardness: 7
Specific gravity: 2.65
Crystal system: trigonal
Crystal shape: hexagonal pyramids and prisms
Chemical structure: SiO_2 silicon dioxide
Natural formations: in hydrothermal and pegmatite sites, in clefts and in hollow spaces in volcanic rock.
Major deposits: Brazil (Minas Gerais); Madagascar; Sri Lanka; Uruguay; Morocco; Zambia

APATITE

Blue apatite is almost unknown in the jewellery trade because of its lack of hardness and is rarely mentioned in the historical literature on gems. However, it has its devotees and among them is much liked for its intense blue colour and transparency.

Healing properties: helps with eye complaints and flu-like infections.

Astrology: Sagittarius; strengthens the emotional area.

Name: Apatite
Group: Apatite
Colour: violet; blue; greenish yellow; pink
Mohs scale hardness: 5
Specific gravity: 3.18 (plus or minus 0.02)
Crystal system: hexagonal
Crystal shape: short and long columns of six-sided prisms
Chemical structure: Ca_5 (F, Cl, OH) $[PO_4]_3$ calcium phosphate
Natural formations: as component of magmatites, pegmatite and volcanic clefts; as druse hollows within metamorphic rocks.
Major deposits: Sri Lanka; Myanmar (Burma); India; Mexico; Brazil; Canada

AQUAMARINE

According to an old legend, aquamarine – or blue beryl – originates in the "the tiny treasure chests of mermaids".

The psychotropic effect of aquamarine has been known in crystal therapy for a long time and it is still employed to calm aggression and help with depression. It is has also been used for treating nervous illnesses and gland disturbance. Its "harmonising" effect induces in its wearer a sense of natural equilibrium, along with greater sensitivity and an awareness of the charisma of others.

Aquamarine is generally considered in astrology to be the crystal of love for the Aquarian. It is therefore believed to encourage friendships and love relationships. It is said to warn the Aquarian of danger.

See also Beryl.

Healing properties: Helps with nervous complaints and disturbances of the glands.

Astrology: Aquarius; strengthens friendships and love, warns of danger. Libra; helps with making decisions and strengthens willpower.

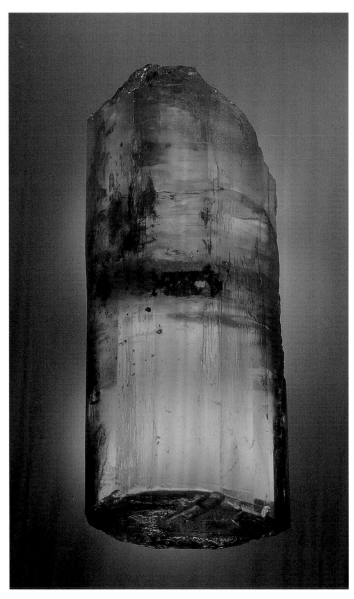

Aquamarine; Brazil

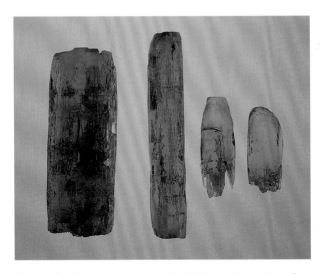

Various beryls; aquamarine variety. Minas Gerais, Brazil

Name: aquamarine
Group: beryl
Colour: greenish blue; pale to deep blue
Mohs scale hardness: 7.5–8
Specific gravity: 2.67–2.71
Crystal system: hexagonal
Crystal shape: six-sided prisms consisting of long columns
Chemical structure: $Al_2Be_3 (Si_6O_{18})$; aluminium beryllium silicate
Natural formations: in pegmatites
Major deposits: Brazil; Madagascar; Russia (Urals); Nigeria; USA

BERYL

This gem was highly prized, even in ancient Mesopotamia from where it entered the culture of ancient Israel. It was here that the mythical status of beryl evolved and where it was revered as a magical gem by the ancient Hebrews and cited as being "in the eighth position in the foundation walls of the New Jerusalem".

Beryl had an important role in the medieval healing arts, not least in its polished state as spectacles, with Brille as the German word for spectacles being derived from "beryl".

Konrad von Megenberg wrote about the healing properties of this gem in the Middle Ages: "I is said, this crystal helps with the throat infection called "angina". The glands, which are caused to swell up because of bad juices in the throat, are driven away if the throat is rubbed with the crystal, especially in the initial stages of infection. This crystal is also able to rekindle love between a married couple, and also bestows upon the wearer an excellent reputation."

Green beryl is also said to heal eye diseases and cure liver complaints.

In astrology, beryl is considered to be the "tireless warning crystal" and is believed to enhance the positive influence of Mercury. Carrying or wearing beryl at all times is recommended as a "protector" on long journeys. Beryl is especially suitable for Geminis, as it is believed to ensure a firm circle of friends. Furthermore, only the very mentally alert Gemini is believed to be able to be fully aware of certain warnings signs evident through the powers of beryl.

Healing properties: treating eye diseases and liver complaints; also helpful with mental, spiritual, psychological and physical exhaustion.

Astrology: Gemini; a tireless warning crystal; the crystal of friendships.

Name: beryl
Group: beryl
Colour: colourless; golden yellow; yellow-green
Mohs scale hardness: 7.5-8

Specific gravity: 2.65 –2.75
Crystal system: hexagonal
Crystal shape: six-sided prisms, with long columns
Chemical structure: $Al_2Be_3[Si_6O_{18}]$ aluminium-beryllium silicate
Natural formations: in pegmatites and their surroundings; in biotite-slate and hydrothermal gangues.
Major deposits: Brazil; Madagascar; Pakistan; Russia.

CARNELIAN

"A talisman made of carnelian brings luck and well being to believers."

Goethe

Carnelian is one of the oldest of decorative gems. The ancient Egyptian pharaohs liked to adorn themselves with it and many carnelian amulets have been discovered in their tombs. Such amulets were part of the "magical armour", which was thought to protect the deceased wearer in the "Life Beyond". The famous Egyptian *Book of the Dead* tells us how the carnelian gem was held in high esteem among the pharaonic culture. It continued to have a high status too in later periods of classical antiquity, where the Greeks and Romans revered it as a decorative gem and magical stone.

Carnelian is red chalcedony, although its colour may range from yellowish-red to reddish-brown. It has been suggested that the name was derived from the Latin word carnis, "flesh", i. e. so that the name carnelian might have meant something like "flesh-red stone". However, it seems much more likely that the name comes from the cornelian cherry, Cornus mas, which the Romans called corneolus.

Because of its colour, carnelian occupied a special place in the treatment of blood diseases and circulation problems. It was also regularly in the Middle Ages to staunch bleeding; and Hildegard von Bingen wrote about this effect as follows:

"Carnelian is more akin to warm air than to cold air and is found in sand. If someone has blood flowing from the nose, warm up some wine and lay the carnelian in it, then let the patient drink thereof and the blood will cease to flow."

In crystal therapy, carnelian is also believed to be helpful against rheumatism. Viewed astrologically, it is the "stone of renewal" and is particularly important to those with the birth sign of Taurus.

Healing effects: in treating rheumatism and circulation problems (especially high blood pressure); also effective in cases of sleeplessness.

Astrology: Taurus; stone of renewal. Aries; strengthens willpower.

Name: carnelian
Group: quartz
Colour: flesh-pink to brownish-red; blood red to yellowish
Mohs hardness: 7
Specific gravity: 2.6
Crystal system: trigonal
Crystal shape: fine fibrous aggregate
Chemical structure: SiO_2 silicon dioxide
Natural formation: in vulcanite rocks
Major deposits: India; Brazil; North Africa; Russia (Siberia); Japan.

CHALCEDONY

Chalcedony was especially admired in antiquity as a material for use in creating decorative gems. Similarly, in Tibet, it was the symbol of the lotus flower, being both pure and translucent, and was believed to have the power to create a deeper self-awareness and even to protect the wearer from attempts at hypnosis. For these reasons, it has been worn for many thousands of years as a talisman to protect against weakness of character, depression and discontent. It was believed to help in retaining and maintaining physical strength and to drive away melancholy.

In the Middle Ages, it was often used as a healing crystal – and Hildegard von Bingen believed that it was formed at sunset, when the air still retains some slight warmth from the day. She considered too that chalcedony protected the wearer from anger and would bestow on the wearer a "peaceful, calm, quiet and amicable nature". Further, it was said that if one breathed on the crystal and touched it with the tongue, one could become more eloquent. It was also credited as a way of healing gall bladder complaints and gout, offering protection from fevers and making its wearer victorious in war.

Chalcedony is now the accepted, comprehensive term for microcrystalline, extremely fine-veined quartz of various different colours, and is supposed to be especially lucky for Cancerians; it is said that chalcedony strengthens the native's emotions and enhances his intuitive facilities.

Healing effects: eases fevers and high temperatures; heals suppurating wounds.

Astrology: Cancer; a lucky stone that boosts the emotions. Sagittarius; provides protection on journeys.

Name: chalcedony
Group: quartz
Colour: blue; bluish-whitish-grey
Mohs hardness: 7
Specific gravity: 2.58–2.64
Crystal system: trigonal
Crystal shape: fibrous aggregate
Chemical structure: SiO_2 silicon dioxide
Natural formation: exuded out of hot, aqueous solutions; also occurs in sedimentary rocks and is found in the form of clumps, as infilling of cracks or in clefts.
Major natural deposits: Brazil; Uruguay; India; Madagascar; USA; Namibia.

CHRYSOBERYL

It was Pliny who first used the name "chrysoberyl" for the yellow or golden beryl, the name being derived from the Greek chrysos, "gold". However, by careful analysis, the German geologist A. G. Werner (1750-1817) established that it was an entirely new mineral, and not any a form of beryl at all.

Because of its golden colour, chrysoberyl was, in the past, associated with wealth. However, as it had a more greenish shade, it was also believed to be effective in the healing of eye diseases and to relieve its wearer from the symptoms of asthma.

Healing effects: treating asthma and eye diseases
Astrology: Leo; bestows confidence and optimism

Name: chrysoberyl
Group: chrysoberyl
Colour: light yellow; golden yellow; yellow; yellowish-green; brownish; greenish-brown
Mohs hardness: 8.5
Specific gravity: 3.7–3.72
Crystal system: prismatic columns
Crystal shape: rhombic
Chemical structure: Al_2 (BeO_4) beryllium aluminate
Natural formation: in granites, pegmatites, mica-containing slate and in alluvial deposits.
Major deposits: Sri Lanka; Brazil; Zimbabwe; Madagascar; Russia (Urals).

CHRYSOPRASE

The name is derived from the Greek word meaning "golden leek"; and in antiquity it was thus described as a green crystal with a propensity towards a golden colour. Similarly, in the Middle Ages, it was described as being "green with a golden drop". The Ancient Egyptians considered that it had magical, healing powers "against the blackish Aspis" (presumed to be the bite of an asp), as the ancient historian Psellus noted in one of the very earliest lapidaries, the Orphic Lithika. Psellus also maintained that chrysoprase ensured better vision for the wearer and could help with stomach pains and swelling if worn around the wrist.

Hildegard von Bingen recorded that chrysoprase was created after sunset and thereby had night-time powers, especially around the time of the half-Moon. It was also said to help with alleviating the pain of gout and could calm feelings of anger and excitement. The most important deposits of chrysoprase were found near Frankenstein in Silesia and, in the fourteenth century, it provided the material for decoration in the famous chapel of Saint Wenceslas in Prague.

Chrysoprase is also said to have a calming effect and will ensure a steady blood circulation in the wearer. Furthermore, it is considered beneficial in any glandular disorders and helps with bleeding and childbirth. Those in the sign of Cancer are supposed to benefit from it by way of their unconscious being revealed with an associated "sharpening of the wits"!

Healing effects: Stabilises the circulation and calms the nerves; also good for treating glandular problems and diseases.

Astrology: Cancer; liberates the unconscious, enhances overall awareness and wits. Capricorn; boosts natural spontaneity.

Name: chrysoprase
Group: quartz
Colour: whitish–green; apple green
Mohs hardness: 7
Specific gravity: 2.6
Crystal system: trigonal
Crystal shape: micro-crystalline aggregate
Chemical structure: SiO_2; silicon dioxide
Natural formation: from eroded deposits, as clumps and infillings of cracks
Major deposits: Australia (Queensland), Brazil; India; Poland (Silesia).

CITRINE

The name of this yellow crystal derives from Medieval Latin and means "the colour of lemons". Genuine citrine is quite rare. In fact, most citrine crystals available in the gem trade are usually smoky quartz that has been "re-coloured" by heat treatment; or can even be amethysts that display reddish-brown shades of colour. This crystal is also sold commercially as "Madeira" or "Golden Topaz".

Healing effects: said to be skin cleansing and "cheering"; alleviates diabetes and glandular disorders.

Astrology: promotes optimism in Geminis and (as golden yellow citrine) is also a lucky crystal for Leos and Virgos in professional ventures.

Name: citrine
Group: quartz
Colour: lemon yellow through to golden brown (the artificial citrine-colouring of heated amethyst).
Mohs hardness: 7
Specific gravity: 2.65
Crystal system: trigonal
Crystal shape: six-sided pyramids; sometimes with prisms
Chemical structure: SiO_2 silicon dioxide
Natural formation: in granites and pegmatites
Major deposits: Brazil; Madagascar; France; Russia; Spain.

CORAL

In Ancient Egypt, the dead were given red coral to act as magical protection on their "journey to the Beyond", as its blood-like colour earned it the reputation of being able to ward off evil on the fateful journey. Perforated coral branches have been found in Gallo-Roman tombs and the Palaeolithic peoples also covered their dead with red chalk from the so-called "raddle stones".

Corals form naturally in the world's warmer seas, being the tiny skeletons of marine polyps, however, it was the shape and colour that helped coral obtain its mysterious reputation, with it often being worn as an amulet. According to Greek mythology, corals were thought to be "drops of blood", which had petrified in the sea after Perseus had hacked off the head of the Gorgon, Medusa.

This legend was the origin of the use of coral as a healing agent – blood was associated with life, and the Gorgon's head with the "evil eye". Children often had chains of coral hung about their necks in order to protect their lives and encourage growth.

Zoroaster, the Persian religious reformer, praised the healing power of coral and was of the opinion that it was popularly used in jewellery because it would protect the wearer against illness and magic. These sorts of beliefs about coral also influenced the West, where coral amulets enjoyed great popularity in the Renaissance, especially in Italy. Coral jewellery is also to be seen in religious paintings and depictions of saints. This fact has never been fully explained, although it does seem to add to the earlier concepts of coral being regarded as being a very special mineral, as some form of material sacra. The historian Paracelsus emphasied the fact that coral protected the wearer from any kind of magic, thereby confirming its frequent uses as amulets and talismans, and King Ferdinand I of Naples (1479-1516) was said always to have had a branch of coral about his person as protection against the "evil eye".

Coral is regarded highly in other cultures too. For example, it is sacred to peoples as varied as the Tibetans and Native American Navaho.

In the magic arts, it is said that coral can turn sorrow into joy and protect the wearer generally from depression, melancholia and hypochondria. Further, it was also believed to guard against fire and drought, and to make fields particularly fertile. As a result, it was often strewn out when sowing seed.

Coral was reputed to have a special effect as a talisman for dancers. It was also believed (as Paracelsus noted) to encourage the love of truth, to protect the wearer from fear and temptation by the Devil, ward off lightning and render poisons ineffective.

It is in its red form that coral is considered to bestow the most potent magical powers. On the Indonesian island of Java, so-called akabar bracelets have been made from it for more than two thousand years, and are said to protect the wearer from poisons and to heal cases of gout.

In the healing arts, it is said that coral aids digestion and can heal extraneous growths such as warts, ulcers and boils. It is also used to treat eye diseases, minor deafness, bone disease and pains in the extremities, especially in children. When used in this way, it is also believed to indicate its curing of any illness in the wearer by becoming paler in colour.

In astrology, red coral is thought to bring luck to Scorpios by reducing the sign's inherent eccentric tendencies. In this way, it is said that a Scorpio can tone down cravings for control and adopt a more reasoned and thoughtful approach to life.

Healing effects: treating bone diseases, ulcers and colic.

Astrology: Scorpio; lucky stone. Libra: sharpens the intellect. Capricorn (black coral); enhances creativity.

Name: coral

Group: -

Colour: delicate pink through dark blood-red; black; blue

Mohs hardness: 3 - 4

Specific gravity: 2.6–2.7 (black coral 1.34 – 1.46)

Crystal system: trigonal

Crystal shape: micro-crystalline

Chemical structure: $CaCO_3$ calcium carbonate, from the skeletal deposits of minute marine organisms (polyps).

Natural formation: Corals are found in the seas in the forms of reefs, atolls and banks with multi-branching structures. The miniscule polyps that live in tiny cavities and exude a chalky substance, causing the gradual build-up of the coral formations.

Major deposits: the coasts of the western Mediterranean, the Bay of Biscay, the Canary Islands, the Malayan archipelago, north-east cost of Australia and the Red Sea.

DIAMOND

Because of its great hardness (the hardest of all minerals at Mohs 10), its unique refraction of light and ability to scatter colour, the diamond is considered to be the "king of precious stones" - as the famous Roman writer Pliny said:

"It was the most valuable among all human possessions...and it was for a long time only known to queens, and not even to many of them either".

Diamonds were first brought to Europe from India via the trading caravans. "Fragments of eternity" is a term still used for the diamond by Indians to this day. Many legends surround the famous Indian diamonds, which often have a most incredible transparency, and were given equally magnificent names such as the "Great Moghul" and the "Nizam".

Astonishingly, the classical opinion that the diamond could be broken only "by the blood of the ram", persisted into the Middle Ages. Indeed up until the late middle Ages, the only known way of working and enhancing diamonds was to polish the naturally occurring surfaces of the gem. It was not until the cutting and polishing of diamonds into brilliant gems - a process invented by Louis van Berquen in 1456 - that the unique spectacular optical qualities of the diamond could be displayed and enjoyed to their full effect.

Because of its unique transparency and purity, the diamond was perceived religiously, and connected, with the concept of the "divine glory on Earth". Based on its very highly prized qualities, the diamond was often employed in healing and in magical medicine. For centuries - at least, for those who could afford it - diamond powder served as a treatment against various illnesses, especially those of the stomach and intestines. A well-known case is that of Pope Clement VII; who (allegedly) took pulverised diamonds "to a value of 40,000 ducats" in order to cure his stomach complaint.

Even in the twentieth century, the unique status of the diamond has been lauded in popular culture in such book, film and song titles as "Diamonds Are Forever" and "Diamonds Are A Girl's Best Friend".

In astrology, the diamond is classed as a providential stone of the very first order. It is supposed to bestow vital energy and willpower. Anyone who has these characteristics, such as Leos – whose zodiacal crystal is the diamond - should be careful. This is a gem that may (allegedly) tempt one into unmediated, ill-advised and precipitous decisions!

However, for many Leos, diamonds also have a very positive aspect and are said to help one realise or achieve in a diligent way any ambitions worthy of overall admiration. Thus, the diamond is said to give a Leo the possibility of standing by and supporting those who are blamelessly weak or helpless. In addition, it is said to bestow great powers of resistance to bad influences and warns its wearer of the insincerity of others.

For a Virgo, yellow diamonds are recommended. Those born under this sign are often of a rather analytical intellect and are supposed to gain an "emotional dimension" through the influence of a diamond, enhancing the inherent, positive attitude found in Virgos.

Healing effects: use to help with epilepsy, glandular problems and fevers.

Astrology: Leo; a lucky stone that boosts compassion. Virgo; fortifies a positive attitude to life.

Name: diamond
Group: -
Colour: colourless; yellowish; brown; greenish; bluish; reddish and black
Mohs hardness: 10
Specific gravity: 3.47–3.55
Crystal system: cubic
Crystal shape: usually octahedrons and cubes
Chemical structure: C; crystalline carbon

Natural formation: in volcanic pipes often containing diamond-bearing rock called kimberlite. Diamonds are created at a temperature of around 1100–1300 degrees Celsius and under great pressure.

Major deposits: in primary and secondary deposits in Africa, India, Brazil and Siberia.

EMERALD

The first emeralds were dug up near the Red Sea around 2000 BC. They are believed to be at least one source of the immeasurable wealth of the pharaohs of that period. The ancient Egyptians called the emerald the "stone of lovers" and dedicated it to the goddess Isis.

It was held in equally high regard centuries later, as indicated in the thirteenth-century writing of Barthlomaeus Angaelicus:

"The emerald is a noble gem, and its colour is as green as the cool depths of the sea in a clear brilliant sky and sunny weather. It is one of the best among precious gems and the most worthy of adorning a royal hand."

Goethe too was also fascinated by the emerald. For example, he compared the character of Ottilie to the emerald in his work *Wahlverwandschaften*.

On the other side of the world, among the pre-Columbian Inca civilisation of South America, the emerald was a revered as an important gem for decorative jewellery and was used in adorning temples. Then, the Spanish conquistadors Hernan Cortez and Gonzalo Pizarro robbed the Incas of these gems and brought them back to Europe. To this day, many of the most famously known emeralds came from these looted treasures.

The emerald has been a highly valued crystal ever since its first discovery. It was used mainly as a healing agent for eye complaints - to the extent that, in antiquity, small beads of emerald were actually placed in the corners of affected eyes.

The Roman historian Pliny, wrote as follows about the healing effects of the emerald: "If the eyes are weakened through too much effort, they will be revived through gazing at the emerald, and the eyes of a stone cutter can benefit no more than doing thus, as the gems gentle green colour drives away exhaustion".

Later, in the Middle Ages, the gem was used for treating headaches; the patient was supposed to breathe on the gem, and then stroke it across the temples and the forehead.

Astrologically, the emerald is assigned to the sign of Cancer as an "emblem of hope". It is supposed to ensure harmony and open-mindedness.

Healing effects: effective against bacterial infections, headaches and fevers.

Astrology: Cancer; a symbol of hope; confers inner harmony. Virgo (trapiche emerald); a lucky stone.

Name: emerald

Group: beryl

Colours: emerald-green; light green; green; dark green

Mohs hardness: 7.5 – 8

Specific gravity: 2.67 – 2.78

Crystal system: hexagonal

Crystal shape: six-sided prisms

Chemical structure: Al_2Be_3 (Si_6O_{18}) aluminium beryllium silicate; green colouration from admixtures of chromium

Natural formation: in metamorphic rocks (biotite slates) and hydrothermal gangues

Major deposits: Columbia; Russia (Urals); Brazil; Pakistan; India; Austria (Habach Valley)

FALCON'S EYE

See TIGER'S EYE for History, Healing effects and Astrology

Name: Falcon's Eye

Group: quartz

Colour: dark blue-grey to blue-green

Mohs hardness: 7
Specific gravity: 2.65
Crystal system: trigonal
Crystal shape: pseudo-morphous
Chemical structure: SiO_2 silicon dioxide
Natural formation: as inclusions in quartz and occasionally within the fibres of the blue asbestos form known as crocidolite.

FIRE OPAL
See OPAL for history, healing effects and astrology.

Name: fire opal
Colour: fiery red; orange; amber coloured
Mohs hardness: 5.5 – 6.5
Specific gravity: 2.1
Crystal system: amorphous
Crystal shape: kidney-shaped aggregates, like bunches of grapes
Chemical structure: SiO_2; aqueous formations of silicon dioxide
Natural formation: in cracks and hollow spaces within volcanic rock
Major deposits: Mexico; Brazil; Turkey.

GARNET

> "Noble garnet... the new day.
> The freshness of life and the morning
> [have] sprinkled morning dew...
> across all the fields of the future."
> Jean Paul

The garnet was well known to the Romans and referred to by them as carbunculus almandious. Garnets also turn up regularly in the histories of other cultures; for example the Jewish *Talmud* tells us that Noah's Ark was illuminated by a single, large garnet.

It is a sacred stone of Buddhism; and, because of its colour, is associated in Hindu tradition with the kundalini fire, the holy fire of transformation, so that it continues to have a high degree of religious meaning in India.

Since its very earliest historical references, garnet has always been considered a protective crystal. It was given to friends to be worn as an amulet on dangerous or difficult journeys. Later, in the Middle Ages, it had the reputation of being the magical "carbuncle stone", taken by knights on the Crusades in order to render themselves invulnerable. A famous garnet, known as "the Wise One", used to be part of the old crown of the German Ottonian emperors.

The word garnet itself stems from the Latin granatus, 'grainy'. It is also possible that the origin of the name comes from the pomegranate tree, the fruit and flowers of which are reminiscent of the colour of garnet. As is so often the case in crystal therapy, the colour of the gem also gives an indication for its use. Thus, the garnet was used for centuries for blood/circulation indications, as a sixteenth-century doctor noted:

"Garnet makes fresh blood...makes the heart glad and inspires confidence".

In the eighteenth century, the garnet was included as one of the five major medical crystals generally known to medicine. Thus, we find the following in Zedler's *Realenzyklopädie*:

"Garnets are reputed to have the power to strengthen the heart, to regulate a too fast pulse, drive away melancholy, and to withstand poison. Thus they serve to staunch bleeding and prevent diarrhoea; a garnet is ground down very finely on a stone; then give the patient from 10 grains to one scruple. Some also make a tincture of it, which is reputed to be good against the red dysentery."

In addition, the garnet is still presumed in crystal therapy to be a supplier of natural energy in sexual health, no other crystal (except coral) can surpass the garnet in its alleged ability to ward off bad luck or disaster. In folk remedies, its red colour thus still plays an important role in this respect.

In astrology, garnet is believed specifically to give an Ariean additional self-confidence and to maintain the "glow of friendship".

Healing effects: maintains a good circulation; soothes pain.

Astrology: Aries; strengthens self-confidence

The following crystals, among others, also belong to the garnet group:

Name: almandine
Group: garnet
Colour: red
Mohs hardness: 6.5 – 7.5
Specific gravity: c. 4.2
Crystal system: cubic
Crystal shape: isometric
Chemical structure: $Fe_3 Al_2 [SiO_4]_3$ iron (ferric) aluminium silicate
Natural formation: in regional metamorphic rocks, such as gneiss and mica slates
Major deposits: Sri Lanka; Brazil; India; Sweden; Alaska; Afghanistan; Madagascar.

Name: pyrope
Group: garnet
Colour: red
Mohs hardness: 6.5 – 7.5
Specific gravity: 3.5
Crystal system: cubic
Crystal shape: isometric
Chemical structure: Mg3Al2 [SiO4]3 magnesium aluminium silicate
Natural formation: derived from alakaline serpentines
Major natural deposits: Czech Republic; South Africa; Australia.

Name: spessartine
Group: garnet

Colour: orange to reddish brown
Mohs hardness: 6.5 – 7.5
Specific gravity: 4.12 – 4.2
Crystal system: cubic
Crystal shape: isometric
Chemical structure: $Mn_3Al_2(SiO_4)_3$ manganese aluminium silicate
Natuaral formation: in granites and pegmatite; also in metamorphic rocks
Major deposits: Madagascar; Sri Lanka; Canada; USA; Brazil; Russia

HAEMATITE

Even the ancient Egyptians placed amulets of haematite in the tombs of their dead. These were laid under the head of the deceased, in order to ease his passage into the Otherworld. Hematite amulets were also found among the "magical armour" of Tutankhamun.

In the *Orphic Lithica*, one of the most important lapidaries of antiquity, the creation of haematite was explained as follows: "When once Uranus, who was mutilated by the bloody hands of Kronos, bent his mighty chest over the Earth, drops of his divine blood ran down onto the clods of earth and solidified in the Sun's heat; no wonder then that this congealed blood contains such healing powers against eye diseases, so that mortals should not be deprived of the sight of the beautiful Heavens."

It was not only eye diseases that were thought to be cured by hematite, for it was also ascribed a blood-staunching effect from the very earliest times. It may be this association, or the fact that some forms show a red-coloured streak that gave the mineral its names. Whatever, the magical effect of hematite is also mentioned time and again throughout history. In the Orient it was said it could protect beautiful maidens from the influence of the "evil eye".

It also had great significance in early metal working, being a principle ore of iron. Astrologically, even in the ancient Orient, haematite was assigned to Mars and thus to the sign of Scorpio.

Healing effects: blood staunching and protection against eye diseases.

Astrology: Scorpio; warns, through dreams, of imminent dangers.

Name: haematite (ferric oxide; iron glance; kidney stone)
Group: -
Colour: blackish-brown; brownish red
Mohs hardness: 5.5 – 6.5
Specific gravity: 4.9 – 5.3
Crystal system: trigonal
Crystal shape: nodules, often kidney-shaped
Chemical structure: Fe_2O_3 iron (ferric) oxide
Natural formation: as accompanying mineral in volcanic rock, often in lava; in pegmatites and in hydrothermal gangues.
Major natural deposits: USA; Canada; Switzerland; Italy; British Isles.

INDIGOLITH
(See TOURMALINE for history, healing effects and astrology)

Name: indigolith
Group: tourmaline
Colour: all shades of blue
Mohs hardness: 7 – 7.5
Specific gravity: 3.0 – 3.3
Crystal system: trigonal
Crystal shape: usually long-stretched prisms
Chemical structure: $(Na, Li, Ca) (Fe, Mg, Mn, Al)_3/Al_6 [(OH)_4 /(Bo_3)_3 /Si_6O_{18}]$
Natural formation: in pegmatites
Major deposits: Brazil; Madagascar; Namibia

JASPER

Even in ancient times, jasper was counted among the most precious of gems by the cultures of the time. For example, it played a major part in the magical Egyptian art of gem cutting called glyptics.

It also became very popular among the Greeks and Romans, as a crystal for amulets and seals, as it was believed to be able to conjure up rain and drive away demons or wild animals. It was even believed to help orators to success and power. The ancient Hebrews also afforded jasper a considerable reputation, as Konrad von Megenberg noted: "...among the gems of Aaron's breastplate of office it occupied the last position, and among the foundation stones of the New Jerusalem the first position."

He also mentions jasper as a green stone in the context of the Book of Revelation, where it is described as belonging among the twelve stones, "...which are called the chosen ones and which were seen by [Saint] John. The green colour is interspersed with small red dots... If it is worn by a chaste person, he will be safe from fevers and dropsy. It also helps women in labour and ensures, if it has been given the 'blessing of stones', that the wearer is safe and comfortable; it also drives away unpleasant or evil visions in dreams..."

In crystal therapy, it was heliotrope among the jasper group that was regarded as being of the greatest importance. In 1583, Leonhard Thurneysser ascribed, in his *Onomasticum* (a form of medieval dictionary), a beneficial effect of jasper in cases of epilepsy. It was also said to have the ability to staunch blood and close wounds.

Jasper is supposed to ensure good order in the spiritual life of anyone born under Aries. It is also believed to bestow luck on the wearer in the conduct of business affairs.

Healing effects: treating epilepsy and bladder problems; also said to have a blood-staunching property.

Astrology: Aries and Virgo; a lucky stone.

Name: jasper
Group: quartz

Colour: many shades of colour; usually streaky or patchy, red, brown, yellow, green

Mohs hardness: 6.57

Specific gravity: 2.5 - 2.9

Crystal system: trigonal

Crystal shape: micro-crystalline, grainy aggregate

Chemical structure: SiO_2; silicon oxide

Natural formation: in eroded rock or in hydrothermal solutions, which occur as infillings of cracks and hollow spaces in various types of rock.

Major deposits: India; Russia; France; Germany; Egypt; USA.

LABRADORITE

Labradorite was first described at the end of the eighteenth century. Its name derives from Labrador, the north-eastern Canadian peninsula where it was first found. It is renowned for its unmistakable range of colour. Individual, closely packed layers (lamellae) of potassium feldspar create a fantastic display of colours, which can range through the whole spectrum – though the dominant colours tend to be blue and green.

Healing effects: treating circulation problems and rheumatism.

Astrology: Aquarius; encourages the imagination.

Name: labradorite (or spectrolith)

Group: feldspar group

Colour: smoky grey; dark grey to greyish-black; bluish with a play of different hues

Mohs hardness: 6 - 6.5

Specific gravity: 2.70 (plus or minus 0.05)

Crystal system: triclinic

Crystal shape: sheet-like prisms ; mostly coarse aggregates

Chemical structure: $Na[AlSi_3O_8]/Ca[Al_2Si_2O_8]$; sodium calcium aluminium silicate crystal mixture

Natural formation: occurs in basal (alkaline) magmatites

Natural deposits: Finland; Russia; USA; Canada; Madagascar; Australia

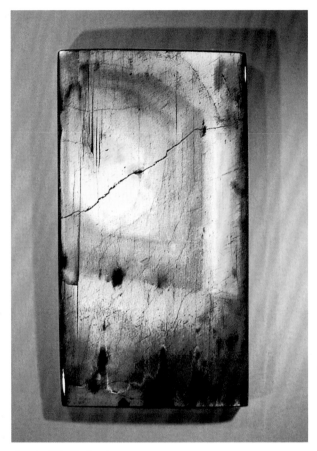

Spectrolith, Finland

LAPIS LAZULI

Lapis lazuli is an ultramarine-coloured compound thought to be one of the first precious gems worked by our ancestors into items of decorative jewellery. Mesopotamian chains of lapis lazuli were found in the royal tombs at the ancient city of Ur on the River Euphrates, along with gold flowers, which had been inlaid with the gem. However, the oldest known site of discovered lapis lazuli jewellery lies in the Hindukush Mountains of Afghanistan.

It also had an important function in South and Central American indigenous cultures, especially for use within sacred rites. In addition, in the Far East, polished lapis lazuli plaques and panels – with their sprinklings of pyrite grains reminiscent of stars in the night sky –led to the mineral being assigned magical qualities and caused it to be revered as sacred, as the stars were believed to guide human fate.

In Ancient Egypt, along the banks of the Nile, whole sculptures of gods were made out of lapis lazuli and it was believed that the gods could live in the sculptures. Also known as lazurite, lapis lazuli served as a symbol of beauty in that culture. Part of the inscription on the so-called Shabaka Stone says the following, of a king's daughter: "Her charms are like those of Anat/Her beauty is like the beauty of Astoreh/Her hair gleams like lapis lazuli."

On his military campaign in Egypt, Napoleon always carried a lapis lazuli scarab that he had taken from a pharaoh's tomb. In fact, lapis lazuli always seems to have exerted a strong attraction on princes and kings. It was the favourite gem of Louis XIV, the French "Sun King", and also of the German Emperor Wilhelm I.

Lapis lazuli was prized for its "virtues" in Christian art. Thus, the painters of the fourteenth century used it to decorate their paintings of the Madonna. The Roman Order of Jesuits owns a globe of lapis lazuli some 60 cm (24 inches) in diameter and depicting the world.

In healing, lapis lazuli is known for its effectiveness against high blood pressure, depression and headaches. It is also supposed to ensure one has refreshing slumber, to be effective against cramp and to strengthen vision. Further, it was also employed in magical medicine in the Middle Ages as a remedy for what was called "four-day fever" and as a calming, protective stone for anxious children. In cosmetics, it was supposed to guarantee an abundance of curly hair!

Astrology attributes lapis lazuli to be a stone of friendship, which encourages relations between people and boosts the self-confidence of the wearer. Sagittarians, in particular, are supposed to be encouraged to turn their intellectual insights and multi-facetted ideas into practical results. Overall, lapis lazuli is said to encourage a sense of community and help one make decisions.

Healing effects: acts against depression, headaches, and neuralgia; eases cramp and is a good sedative.

Astrology: Sagittarius; stone of friendship. Helps in making decisions.

Name: Lapis lazuli (lazurite with mainly calcite and pyrite inclusions)
Group: -
Colours: light blue; blue; bluish violet, often with inclusions of different colours
[calcite (white), pyrite (metallic; shiny like gold)]
Mohs hardness: 5 - 6
Specific gravity: 2.38 - 2.42
Crystal system: cubic
Crystal shape: rarely crystals; usually a grainy mass
Chemical structure: $Na_6Ca_2 [(S, SO_4, Cl_2)_2/Al_6Si_6O_{24}]$ (lazurite) sulphur
sodium aluminium silicate
Natural formation: as a mineral mixture, often with dolomite limestone
Major deposits: Afghanistan; Russia (Lake Baikal); Chile.

MALACHITE

The Ancient Egyptians used malachite, which they extracted from mines between Suez and the Sinai as early as the fourth century BC. The deep green colour and pronounced markings made it much sought after for wearing as an amulet. On the other hand, it was also pulverised and used as eye make-up – yes, eye shadow was used even then – as well as for healing ointments and salves.

Generally speaking, malachite was believed to encourage growth, which meant that it was worn in the form of amulets especially by children and pregnant women. Specifically, in the Alpine regions of Europe, from the sixteenth century onward, so-called "labour-crosses" inlaid with malachite were worn as pregnancy and birth amulets.

Healing effects: Generally growth enhancing and strengthening; blood-staunching and healing; also effective against asthma, poisons, Parkinsonism, multiple sclerosis, and any kind of colic. It was also believed to help with cholera infections and be good for the eyes.

Astrology: believed to be a lucky stone for Capricorns, but is also lucky for Aquarians.

Name: Malachite
Group: -
Colours: light to dark green; usually banded or striped
Mohs hardness: 3.5-4
Specific gravity: 4
Crystal system: monoclinic
Crystal shape: needle-like fibres or fibrous aggregates
Chemical structure: $Cu_2[(OH)_2/CO_3]$ alkaline copper carbonate
Natural formation: in the oxidation zone of copper deposits
Major deposits: Zaire; Russia; Zambia.

MOONSTONE

The name derives from a translation of the Greek-Latin selenitis, in turn the name of the Moon goddess Selene. Later, the Roman historian Pliny recorded the following:

"Selenitis glows in a white, honey-coloured play of light. It contains the image of the Moon and, day by day, reflects the Moon's waxing and waning nature." However, he did go on to add: "If it is really true."

Identifying moonstone specifically in history is not an easy task. Evidence from medieval traditions is all the more complicated, because there is every indication of mistaken identifications and confusion with other crystals. For example, it is said that people who suffered from "the falling sickness" (epilepsy) were supposed to take beverages containing pulverised moonstone, while also being advised to wear it as an amulet.

However, from the end of the eighteenth century onward, progress in mineralogy resulted in a clear identification of moonstone, the term that is now recognised for what are specific types of feldspar in a polished state and displaying a milky-white gleam.

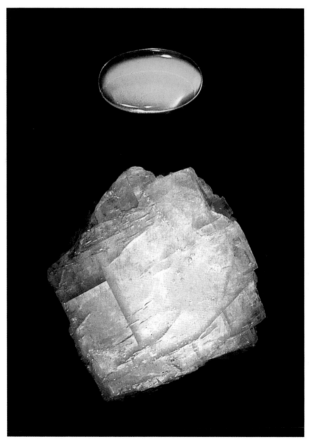

Moonstone, polished; rough and unpolished, Sri Lanka

Nonetheless, moonstone was considered to be a magical gem in nearly all cultures. Some Arab women still sew pieces of it into their clothing, in order to ensure the blessing of many children. In India, the moonstone is regarded as a "dream stone" and is supposed to bring its bearer beautiful dreams.

In crystal therapy, the moonstone is supposed to have a healing effect on the lymph glands and also help women to maintain a proper hormonal balance. Astrologically speaking. Moonstone enhances the ascribed "lunar characteristics" of Cancerians and promotes inner harmony. In addition, dream activity is seemingly stimulated; and enhanced in Cancerians (see above regarding Indian ideas about moonstone). The blue form of moonstone enhances the alleged "intuitive abilities" in Pisceans, as those with this sign of the zodiac are regarded, astrologically, as having tendencies to see the future or become mediums.

Healing effects: treating lymphatic disorders. Can create a proper hormonal balance in women.

Astrology: Cancer; fortifies the "lunar qualities" and ensures inner harmony. Pisces (blue moonstone); boosts natural intuitive ability.

Name: moonstone
Group: feldspar group
Colours: blue; colourless; yellow; silky white to bluish shimmering effect.
Mohs hardness: 6
Specific gravity: 2.5
Crystal system: monoclinic
Crystal shape: prismatic
Chemical structure: K $[AlSi_3O_8]$ potassium aluminium silicate
Natural formation: on pegmatitic gangues with quartz.
Major deposits: Sri Lanka; southern India; Brazil; USA; Madagascar.

MOSS AGATE
See AGATE for History, Healing effects and Astrology

Name: moss agate
Group: quartz group
Colours: colourless with green and reddish brown inclusions
Mohs hardness: 6.5 – 7
Specific gravity: 2.58 – 2.62
Crystal system: trigonal
Crystal shape: micro-crystalline
Chemical structure: SiO_2 silicon dioxide
Natural formation: found within cracks in granites and pegmatites.
Major deposits: India; USA; China.

NEPHRITE
Nephrite was used in many different cultures for the manufacture of weapons and tools. Stone axes made by the Maoris, the Polynesians and pre-Columbian peoples of Central America were all fashioned from nephrite. The latter civilisations in particular used nephrite for their axes that were particularly impressive in the perfection of their shapes and crafting. Initially these axes were used for cult activities but later discovered tools and weapons show them to have become rather more ceremonial in character than for actual sacrifice and the like

In ancient China and East Asia, nephrite was considered to be especially powerful and to have magical meanings. Even though nephrite artefacts are found frequently by archaeologists, it is a mineral that seems always to have been highly valued. Further, engraving or marking with certain symbols appears to have been carried out in the belief that it brought luck to its owner and could ward of any evil influences.

In antiquity, nephrite was especially highly regarded when worn as a heart-shaped amulet or in an image of a god. Amulets like these were thought to protect the wearer from "love magic" in particular. A healing property in connection with kidney problems was also ascribed to nephrite. As a consequence of this, later, medieval physicians gave the stone its own name of lapis nephriticus, or "stone for the kidneys", which soon evolved into "nephrite", from nephros, the Greek for "kidney".

It is no surprise, therefore, that kidney-shaped nephrite pieces are still being worn for their soothing effect and alleviation of kidney disorders. Nephrite is also said to improve eyesight and is generally considered to be a "stone for a long life", which goes back to an ancient Chinese perception. To this day, nephrite amulets in the shape of storks are worn in China. Astrologically, nephrite is said to bring luck, success, and a good reputation; this is especially true for Cancerians who are supposed to wear this stone as a symbol of hope.

Healing effects: in treating kidney complaints. Improves eyesight.

Astrology: Cancer; a symbol of hope.

Name: nephrite

Group: amphibole

Colour: leek green; greenish; grey; white; yellowish; often with patches [spots; flecks;]

Mohs hardness: 5.5 – 6

Specific gravity: 2.95 (plus or minus 0.05)

Crystal system: monoclinic

Crystal shape: finely-fibrous aggregate

Chemical structure: $Ca_2 (Mg, Fe)_5[Si_4O_{11}]_2(OH)_2$ alkaline calcium magnesium iron silicate

Natural formation: in close layers or nest-like deposits between granite and serpentine rock

Major deposits: China; Russia; New Zealand; USA; Canada (British Columbia).

ONYX

Onyx has long been an important stone for jewellery. In Mesopotamia, and later, especially among the Greeks and Romans, it was the preferred gem for making eye amulets. Its power was thought to be enhanced by adding magical inscriptions, as demonstrated in the many examples from archaeological finds from different cultures and historical eras. It was clearly much revered by the Hebrews, as it occurs in several well-known passages of the Pentateuch within the Old Testament.

Polished onyx includes line-like markings that give it an appearance something like a human eye. As a result, it gained a reputation for being an effective therapy against several kinds of eye disease. Thus, Konrad von Megenberg cites it in his *Buch der Natur* (Book of Nature) in 1349 as a means of healing scabies and blurred vision.

Onyx was also much employed as a general agent in strengthening the body. Indeed, all healing processes were believed to be accelerated by applying onyx – for example, using in a pulverised form on suppurating wounds. It was also thought to help with a weak heart and alleviate any problems with blood circulation.

Onyx was considered to be a stone of the magical arts per se. In the Middle Ages, as well as being an aid in meditation, it was even believed that it could bestow upon the wearer the ability to become invisible.

In astrology, onyx is assigned to those with the sign of Capricorn, on whom it was supposed to confer a sense of restraint or caution, secure fidelity in love and protect the wearer from danger. Its effect, however, was thought to be of a somewhat materialistic nature, so that it was supposed to bring luck mainly to those pursuing pecuniary interests.

Curiously, the Ayurveda recommends that the creative, or more "spiritual" types among us should actually refrain from wearing onyx. On the other hand, astrological texts say that onyx – especially the white variety – brings peace to the soul and creates an inner calm. In a complementary way, the black variety helps in attaining a greater seriousness, gravitas, earnestness, greater depth of thought and improved self-control.

Healing effects: heals suppurating wounds and alleviates circulatory complaints.

Astrology: Capricorn; protects from danger and bolsters fidelity in love.

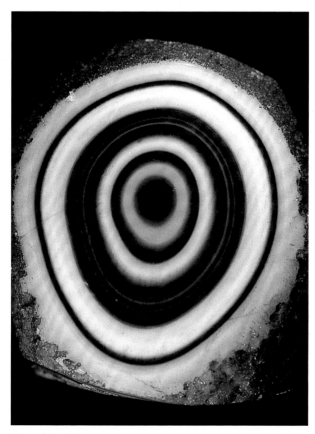

Onyx, Brazil

Name: onyx

Group: quartz

Colours: black (black and white banded variety of chalcedony); often artificially stained in the commercial gem trade; rarely used in natural colours

Mohs hardness: 7

Specific gravity: 2.5 - 2.6
Crystal system: trigonal
Crystal shape: fibrous aggregate
Chemical structure: SiO_2 silicon dioxide
Natural formation: in hollow spaces of volcanic stone of low silicic acid content.
Major deposits: Brazil; India; Madagascar

OPAL

The opal was already highly regarded among the Greeks, whose word for stone (Opalus) provided the origin of the word 'opal'. Pliny compared the opal with other stones and considered that it possessed all of the positive qualities of the other gems put together: "The delicate fire of the carbuncle, the gleaming purple of the amethyst, the splendid sea-green of the emerald, the golden yellow of topaz, the deep blue of the sapphire, so that all the colours shine together in a wonderful mixture".

Many of the truly old opals came from India, where its creation is

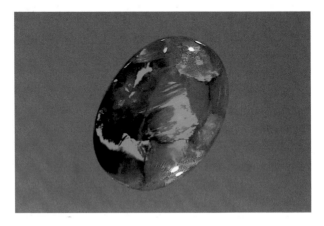

Black Opal, Australia

described in a legend telling of how the gods, Brahma, Vishnu and Shiva were all jealously in love with one goddess. However, The Eternal One, was so angry at such a display of jealousy that he solved the problem by transforming the beautiful goddess into a being made of mist. However, in order that they would not completely lose her in the mist, each of her divine lovers bestowed a colour upon her.

Brahma gave her his wonderful blue; Vishnu gave her the gleam of gold; and Shiva lent her glowing red. But the colourful, misty form was blown apart by the wind. The Eternal One relented and showed mercy, transforming it into a stone – the iridescent precious opal, which unites within itself all the splendid colours of all the gems.

So, in India, the opal is considered to be a bringer of luck and throughout the East it is regarded as a "stone of hope", bringing together the virtues of all the other gems. Elsewhere, in contrast, because of a wide spread superstition of that iridescent things bring bad luck, the opal was for a long time considered to be an unlucky stone.

In astrology, the opal is thought to enhance the positive qualities of Cancerians. It is also recommended for Arians, as it is said to encourage the lat-

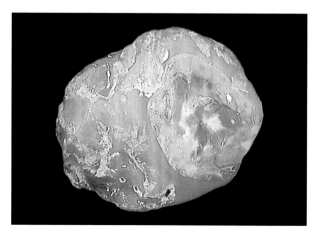

Rough opal, Australia

ter's social commitment. For Scorpios, the black precious opal is believed to drive away depression and night-time fears. Light-coloured opals are generally believed to be calming for the nerves and emotions. Opal and boulder opal are lucky stones for Pisceans.

Healing effects: effective against stomach and intestinal diseases.

Astrology: Cancer; enhances the positive qualities. Aries; (fire opal) alleviates depression. Scorpio; (black precious opal) a lucky stone. Pisces; (boulder opal) provides protection on journeys.

Name: opal, precious opal
Group: opal
Colours: white; grey; blue; green; red; purple; yellow; black; some opalising
Mohs hardness: 5.5 - 6.5
Specific gravity: 1.9 - 2.3
Crystal system: amorphous
Crystal shape: kidney-shaped or grape-bunch-like aggregate
Chemical structure: SiO_2 nH_2O hydrated silicon dioxide containing water
Natural formation: formed by hydrothermal erosion and petrification. Found in hollow spaces within hardened lava.
Major deposits: Australia (in opalising limonite clumps, as so-called boulder opals) Mexico; Hungary (classically); Brazil

PADPARADSHA (SAPPHIRE)

This is a type of sapphire that is also incorrectly known as king topaz or royal topaz. In fact, it is a reddish yellow corundum found in Sri Lanka, hence its exotic sounding name of padparadsha, which means 'lotus flower' in Singhalese. Many wonderful qualities are attributed to this somewhat controversial gemstone, though it is generally supposed to enhance the positive traits of character, protect its wearer on journeys, guard one against false friends and even provide intuitive insights into the future. It is also the stone of wealth and coherent, clear thinking.

Healing effects: well known as a protection against insanity and sleep disturbances; also effective against intestinal pain and exhaustion.

Astrology: the lucky stone of Taurus, whose character traits it is generally believed to enhance; overall, a protective stone.

Name: padparadsha (sapphire)
Group: corundum
Colours: orange–yellow to reddish yellow
Mohs hardness: 9
Specific gravity: 3.99 – 4.0
Crystal system: trigonal
Crystal shape: often barrel-shaped double pyramids
Chemical structure: Al_2O_3 aluminium oxide
Natural formation: in metamorphic rocks and pegmatites; extracted chiefly from alluvial deposits
Major deposits: Sri Lanka

PERIDOT

Peridot, also known as chrysolite or olivine, was already in use as a gem for making jewellery in Egypt in the second millennium BC. In those days, it was obtained mainly from an island in the Red Sea (Zagbargad) where the most important natural deposit still exists. From there, it was brought to Europe by the crusaders, where it often served as a decorative gem for Christian altars. Later, peridots also came to Western Europe through Napoleon's armies. An interesting fact is that this crystal has also been found in some meteorites.

For a long time, the peridot was incorrectly thought to be a topaz. In fact, several famous topazes from history – for example, those described in Exodus as being on the breastplate of Moses' brother Aaron, were actually peridots. At the time of the Greeks and the Romans, who also thought this gem was a topaz, it was considered to be one of the most precious of all.

The evolution of the name is hard to determine, not least because of the change in identification and meaning over time (i.e. confusion in antiquity with the topaz). Consequently, various theories and interpretations exist for possible Greek, Arabic or even Persian origins.

Healing effects: Peridot is considered to be a "tranquilliser", and is said to improve eyesight, help with digestive problems and lift depression.

Astrology: Lends the Gemini confidence, trust and optimism. Believed to be a lucky stone for Librans and beneficial for their health.

Name: Peridot (synonym: chrysolite, olivine)
Group: -
Colours: olive-oil green; bottle green; yellow green to moss green; brownish green
Mohs hardness: 6.5 – 7
Specific gravity: 3.2 – 3.6
Crystal system: rhombic
Crystal shape: short, squat prisms
Chemical structure: $(Mg, Fe)_2 SiO_4$ magnesium iron silicate
Natural formation: as a constituent of alkaline magmatic rocks
Major natural deposits: Red Sea; Myanmar (Burma); Australia; Brazil; USA (Arizona); Pakistan.

PEARL

The pearl, as it is formed naturally within pearl oysters, is actually a product of the animal kingdom. Nevertheless, from time immemorial, it has always been regarded as a precious gem, and so is colloquially accepted as a "mineral".

Pearls were already much loved, precious items among kings and princes of Ancient Egypt, India and Persia. Indeed, the name is most likely derived from an old Persian word. The legendary pearl jewellery of the Queen of Sheba remains famous in religious accounts, as do the pearls in the magical necklace belonging to the Hindu god, Vishnu. Similarly, it is said that Cleopatra greeted her most highly esteemed guests with a special drink containing pulverised pearls of the highest value.

Later, in the Middle Ages and the Renaissance of Europe, the pearl was also highly valued and found only in the courts of princes. More than any other jewel, the pearl inspired poets throughout the ages, who saw in it the symbolic representation of all female beauty. It is not surprising, therefore, that the pearl was dedicated by the Romans to the goddess Venus.

As part of the magical arts, the pearl was believed to possess magnetic powers. It was also believed to be able to warn of future misfortune. For example, Queen Marie Antoinette, while gazing at her pearl necklace, is supposed to have had a vision of her fate some ten years before her execution in the French Revolution.

In crystal therapy, pink pearls are especially prized and used to improve vision, correct poor eyesight and alleviate depression.

From the astrological angle, light-coloured pearls, in particular, are supposed to enhance the Cancerians' sense of aesthetics – whilst black pearls are assigned to those of the sign of Capricorn, and to whom they are supposed be warn of future misfortune or imminent danger.

Healing effects: against eye complaints and depression.

Astrology: Cancer (light-coloured pearls); enhances a sense of aesthetics. Capricorn (black pearls); warns of imminent or future misfortune.

Name: pearl
Group: -
Colours: pink; silver-cream-golden coloured; green; blue; black
Mohs hardness: 3 - 4
Specific gravity: 2.60 - 2.78
Crystal system: -
Crystal shape: -
Chemical structure: 84% - 92% $CaCO_3$ calcium carbonate; 4% - 13% organic substance; 3% - 4% water

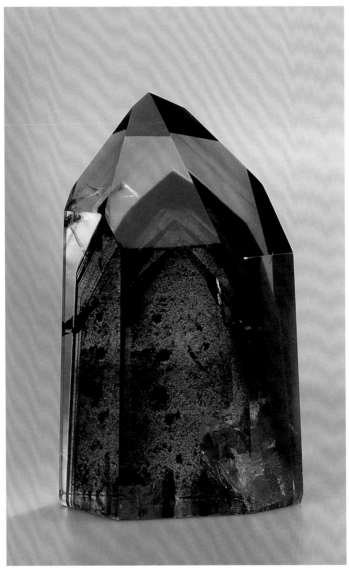

Quartz crystal with phantom formations (coloured with chlorite), Minas Gerais, Brazil.

Natural formation: created through foreign bodies entering between the shell and mantle skin of an oyster. There, in the body of the shell, a defensive reaction occurs, which encapsulates the foreign body in layers of mother-of-pearl (nacre).

Major sources: Persian Gulf; Gulf of Myanmar (Burma); the coasts of Central America and northern Australia.

PYROPE; see GARNET

ROCK CRYSTAL

"Quartz demonstrates its perfection in rock crystal."

Goethe

The idea that rock crystal was fossil ice can be found throughout all of antiquity. Its Greek name of crystallos, meaning "clear ice", supports this view. Even in the Middle Ages, the chemist, Johann Kinkel, assumed that rock crystal was "congealed ice".

Many myths have grown up around this crystal. Mountain peoples, in particular, had countless legends about it and assumed that the mountain spirits had their seats in palaces made of rock crystal. Because of its clarity and transparency, rock crystal was assumed to be the seat of gods of all kinds. Thus, the Emperor Augustus dedicated to a Roman god on the Capitol the largest known rock crystal of his time, one weighing nearly 23 kg (50 lbs).

Rock crystal is considered sacred among Native Americans to this day and newborn babies have a crystal placed in their cradle as a symbol of their connection with the Earth. In Tibet, too, the rock crystal is highly prized; it is supposed to help Tibetan Buddhists to sink into deep meditation and to find the "Path to Enlightenment". In the same way as amethyst, rock crystal is also used as a meditation aid all over the world. People in India

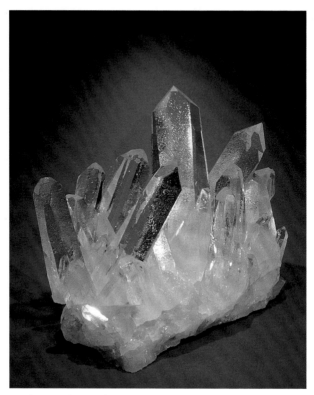

Rock crystal, Brazil.

make "rosaries" of rock crystal, in order to enhance the effectiveness of their prayers. Spheres of crystal, prized for enhancing meditation, are in demand everywhere; and the traditional fortune teller's "crystal ball" has its origins in this practice.

Rock crystal has a long tradition in the healing arts. The Roman historian Pliny described its healing effect and the emperor Nero, whose love of gems was well known, only drank his wine from rock crystal goblets, believing his thirst would be quenched all the quicker.

In the Middle Ages, it was used in folk medicine against thirst and against chilblains. When held up to the Sun, a crystal ball was believed to heal the skin, especially blisters from burns. Rock crystal was also employed for staunching bleeding and for treating complaints linked to the gall bladder; and Hildegard von Bingen recommended that nursing mothers take ground up rock crystal mixed with honey.

The shape of a rock crystal plays an important role in its healing effect. A pyramid shape with a pointed end is especially effective in directing and focusing the crystal's positive energy in a cohesive, targeted manner onto the infected or ailing part of the body. The energy rays were thus believed to enter the body more effectively and ensure "internal harmony". Rock crystal is believed to enhance basic intuition and the ability to concentrate. Especially in Leos, it is also alleged to bestow an ability to see the future.

Healing properties: for skin problems and staunching blood flow.

Astrology: Leo; a meditation crystal that enhances intuition.

Name: rock crystal
Group: quartz
Colour: colourless; usually clear and transparent
Mohs scale hardness: 7
Specific gravity: 2.65
Crystal system: trigonal
Crystal shape: six-sided prisms
Chemical structure: SiO_2; silicon dioxide
Natural formations: in clefts and in druse hollows; in pegmatites and hydrothermal gangues
Major deposits: Brazil (Minas Gerais); the Alps (Austria; Switzerland); Japan; Madagascar; USA (Arkansas)

ROSE QUARTZ

Rose quartz was already an important gem for making jewellery in the Middle Ages, when it was also found in Central Europe, in the Bohemian Forest region, and was used to decorate the Saint Wenceslas Chapel in Prague.

Its name derives from its pale-to-dark pink colour, reminiscent of that of many types of rose. This range of sensual and attractive colours also explains why it was attributed with having healing properties – as the principles of so-called "sympathetic magic" tended to assign gems with red-coloured stones (such as garnets, rubies and carnelians) to the treatment of ailments associated with the blood, e.g. circulation and heart ailments.

It was reputed to have a property of enhancing one's joie de vivre and bring about luck in love. As a result, rose quartz has always been a favourite crystal among young girls and remains so today.

Modern sources include the USA, Sri Lanka and Japan in Asia and Austria and the British Isles in Europe.

Healing effects: treating blood diseases, circulation and heart problems, shingles and related skin diseases; also deemed to be both enlivening and "refreshing".

Astrology: assigned to Taurus and thought to enhance powers of imagination and artistic skills, and bestow luck in love.

Name: rose quartz
Group: quartz
Colours: deep pink to pale pink
Mohs hardness: 7
Specific gravity: 2.65
Crystal system: trigonal
Crystal shape: usually coarse; rarely, as six-sided prisms
Chemical structure: SiO_2 silicon dioxide
Natural formation: in pegmatites
Major natural deposits: Brazil; Madagascar; Germany (Zweisel in Bavaria; USA; Namibia.

RUBELLITE
(See TOURMALINE regarding the history, healing properties and astrology)

Name: rubellite
Group: tourmaline
Colours: pink to red; occasional hints of violet
Mohs hardness: 7 – 7.5
Specific gravity: 3.0 – 3.2
Crystal system: trigonal
Crystal shape: usually as long prisms
Chemical structure: $(Na, Li, Ca) (Fe, Mg, Mn, Al)_3 Al_6 [(OH)_4/(BO_3)_3/SiO_{18}]$
Natural formation: in pegmatites
Major natural deposits: Brazil; Mozambique; Madagascar

RUBY

Because of their colourful variety, the corundum mineral group – crystallised aluminium oxides – are considered to be the "flowers in the kingdom of precious gems". As Aristotle wrote about rubies:

"One is red as pure blood and is called rubinus. That is the best of all".

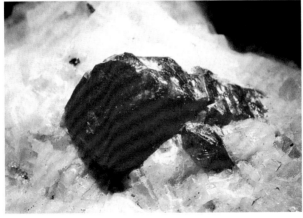

Ruby, Pakistan

This much-lauded gem was royally revered throughout history. Whenever a particularly splendid specimen was found in the East, the local ruler would send high-ranking dignitaries and soldiers, in order to prepare a proper state reception for the jewel. There, in the Orient, this "drop of blood from the heart of Mother Earth" was said to have great healing powers.

The Arab philosopher and physician, Avicenna (980-1037) wrote the following of the ruby: "This is a [well-tempered] stone. It has the unique quality of being able to make the heart happy and to strengthen it. As for the part of the body affected [by it], it is evident that the stone is able to reach the heart through the blood; the closer it is placed to the diseased part of the body, the more effective it is".

In the Middle Ages in Europe, the ruby was worn in order to ward off plague, when it was believed that the gem would turn darker in response to approaching misfortune. This is a conviction that still survives, surprisingly, in certain belief systems.

Ruby was also thought to protect the wearer from nightmares and, astrologically, it is held that the ruby possesses the "original spark of life" – so is considered to be a lucky stone. For Arieans, it is believed to reinforce their natural intuitive abilities and powers of regeneration.

Healing effects: good for treating eye complaints, feverish illnesses and colic; stimulates sexual energy.

Astrology: Aries; strengthens the intuition and regenerates natural energy reserves.

Name: ruby
Group: corundum
Colours: various shades of red
Mohs hardness: 9
Specific gravity: 3.99 – 4.0
Crystal system: trigonal
Crystal shape: six-sided prisms
Chemical structure: Al_2O_3 aluminium oxide

Natural formation: in metamorphic rocks; extracted mainly from alluvial
deposits
Major deposits: Myanmar (Burma); Thailand; Sri Lanka; Tanzania; India;
Vietnam.

SAPPHIRE

> "And when we wish to express ourselves most poetically,
> we compare the sapphire with the clearest blue of the heavens...."
>
> Goethe

The sapphire has always been used as a way to describe the most beautiful
shades of blue, especially that of the heavens. In the *Bible*, the sapphire is
mentioned by the prophet Ezekiel in the Old Testament; and in the New
Testament in Revelation, where the sapphire turns up as one of the foundation stones of the "New Jerusalem".

The images conjured up of sapphires in the *Bible* were further embel-
lished during the Middle Ages by a series of Christian allegories. The sapphire was considered to be the "guiding stone" of emperors and kings, who
fulsomely praised its virtues very widely – not least because of its protective
powers. Indeed, such powers seemed to have been already known in antiquity and Damigeron wrote:

"God bestows great honour on the sapphire. Kings are accustomed to
wearing this gem about their necks, as it provides the most powerful protection".

As a magical gem, it was believed to possess many beneficial qualities.
Hildegard von Bingen was convinced that the sapphire could be employed
successfully against demonic possession. In addition, according to Konrad
von Megenberg, it had the power to endow the wearer with a peaceful dis-
position and to protect from infidelity and hatred. Around the same time, the
sapphire was also believed to cure what was called "the madness of love".

In addition to these qualities, the sapphire was also said to have the power to staunch blood and have other healing powers. It is still applied in modern crystal therapy for fortifying the nervous system and for aiding cases of heart diseases.

See also PADPARADSAHA

Astrologically, it is regarded as being as the "stone of faith" or of "peace of the soul". A light-coloured sapphire is believed to support the overall range of spiritual virtues of the Taurean; but it is also thought to enhance a willingness to explain and discuss matters with others. For Virgo, the yellow form of sapphire is considered to be the gem of protection par excellence.

Healing effects: useful against heart diseases, whooping cough, loss of appetite and blood staunching; fortifies the nervous system.

Astrology: Taurus (light-coloured sapphire); enhances spiritual qualities. Virgo (yellow sapphire); a protective gem. Pisces (blue); bestows confidence and trust. Gemini (yellow); encourages self-confidence. Taurus (light coloured padparadsha); a lucky stone. Libra (star sapphire); a protective stone.

Name: sapphire
Group: corundum
Colours: various shades of blue; colourless; green; pink; yellow; orange
Mohs hardness: 9
Specific gravity: 3.99 – 4.0
Crystal system: trigonal
Crystal shape: often as barrel-shaped double-pyramids
Chemical structure: Al_2O_3 aluminium oxide; the colour is determined by the degree of admixtures of iron and titanium
Natural formation: in basalts, metamorphic rocks and pegmatites.
Major deposits: Australia; Myanmar(Burma); Sri Lanka; Thailand.

SARD

According to classical tradition, this stone was first found in Sardes, a town in Asia Minor, which is also supposed to have given it its name. Another theory says that the old Persian word serd, which means "yellowish red", is the derivation of the name. As descriptions from antiquity credit this gem with this colour, one may assume that the "sard" or "sardius" of ancient texts referred to a reddish form of chalcedony. By extension, the assumption is also that "sard" as mentioned in the Book of Revelation was also "reddish".

However, from the Middle Ages onward, the name carnelian became commonly used for this red gem; and the name "sard" or "sardonyx" was thereafter only used for the brown form of chalcedony.

Healing effects: used against arthritis and rheumatism
Astrology: Scorpio; a lucky stone

Name: sard, sardius or sardonyx
Group: quartz
Colours: red-brown (and brown-white) variety of chalcedony
Mohs hardness: 7
Specific gravity: 2.58 – 2.64
Crystal system: trigonal
Crystal shape: fibrous aggregate
Chemical structure: SiO_2 silicon dioxide
Natural formation: in once-hollow spaces of volcanic rocks, which are low in silicic acid content
Major deposits: Brazil; India; Madagascar.

SPECTROLITH; see LABRADORITE

SPESSARTINE; see GARNET

SPINEL

Most spinels are reddish in colour, but blue, green and black varieties also occur. The name is, presumably, derived from the Greek term for "spark", which probably refers to the red colouration, especially that of the noble and precious varieties of the mineral. In the early Middle Ages, healing powers were attributed to the spinels that were especially associated with various kinds of inflammations. However, spinel was also recommended for its general calming effect and for settling quarrels.

Red spinels were sometimes confused with rubies. This is probably the explanation for the erroneous name of the famous spinel, the "Black Prince's Ruby", which adorns the British State Crown (alongside what is perhaps the second-largest diamond in the world).

Healing effects: used for inflammations of any kind; has a calming effect.

Astrology: dark-blue spinel is the lucky stone of Sagittarians and is supposed to help them particularly in developing their musical talents; red

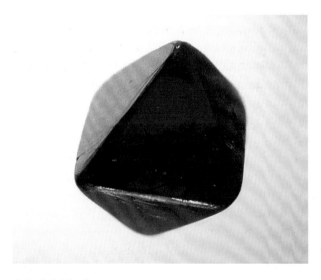

Spinel, Sri Lanka

spinel is assigned to Scorpios, whose emotional character traits it is said to fortify.

Name: spinel
Group: -
Colours: pink, red, violet, yellowish orange, blue, dark green, black
Mohs hardness: 8
Specific gravity: 3.58 – 3.61
Crystal system: cubic
Crystal shape: octahedron
Chemical structure: Mg (Al_2O_4) magnesium aluminium oxide
Natural formation: in magmatites and metamorphic rocks; found in large deposits of alluvial material
Major natural deposits: Myanmar (Burma); Thailand; Sri Lanka; Afghanistan; Brazil; USA (New Jersey).

STAR SAPPHIRE
See SAPPHIRE regarding History, Healing Effects and Astrology

When polished as a cabochon, it displays on its surface the effect of a "moving", six-point star. This consists of three lines that intersect and is caused by fine, parallel hollow channels, which reflect the light in a unique way.

Name: star sapphire
Group: corundum
Colours: blue; grey bluish; black
Mohs hardness: 9
Specific gravity: 3.99 – 4.0
Crystal system: trigonal
Crystal shape: often as barrel-shaped double-pyramids
Chemical structure: Al_2O_3 aluminium oxide; colouration arises from admixtures of iron and/or titanium

Areas of formation: in basalts, metamorphic rocks, exploitation mainly from
alluvial deposits
Major deposits: Australia; Myanmar; Sri Lanka; Thailand.

TANZANITE

A blue, gemstone variety of zoisite that was first found in 1967 in the
Arusha Mine in Tanzania. The original find site is now almost exhausted,
as the gem is very much in demand in the commercial jewellery-making
industry.

Healing effects: no applications known – so far.

Astrology: Sagittarius; nothing specific assigned to date

Name: tanzanite (blue zoisite)
Group: -
Colours: sapphire blue; amethyst violet; bluish violet
Mohs hardness: 6 – 6.5
Specific gravity: 3.35
Crystal system: rhombic
Crystal shape: prismatic, but often multi-faceted; usually banded
Chemical structure: $Ca_2Al_3[O/OH/Si_2O_7]$ calcium aluminium silicate
Areas of formation: in metamorphic rocks
Major deposits: Tanzania.

TIGER'S EYE

Tiger's Eye, Cat's Eye and Falcon's Eye are all related crystals – and all of
them quartzes. When given a particular polishing, they are then reminiscent of the optical effect of animal eyes when reflecting directly incidental
light – a function of the fibrous inclusions within the mineral.

Tiger's eye has been recorded in South Africa ever since the second half
of the nineteenth century. Tiger's eye is a metamorphic form of falcon's eye
and displays, as the name suggests, a yellowish brown colour.

See also FALCON'S EYE
Healing effects: good against asthma and colds; said to "warm the body"
Astrology: Virgo

Name: tiger's eye
Group: quartz
Colours: golden yellow; golden brown
Mohs hardness: 6.5 - 7
Specific gravity: 2.5 - 2.7
Crystal system: trigonal
Crystal shape: fibrous aggregate
Chemical structure: SiO_2 silicon dioxide
Areas of formation: as inclusions in gangues of metamorphic rocks
Major deposits: South Africa; Western Australia.

TOPAZ

The most valuable form of topaz, and also the best known, is the golden topaz. In addition to this yellow-brown form, with its warm, red undertones, there are also light blue, green blue and even colourless types.

Clearly, topaz was known and revered in Old Testament times: "The topaz of Ethiopia shall not equal it" Job 28; 19

Nevertheless, the origin of the name has yet to be clarified. According to tradition, shipwrecked pirates are supposed to have discovered the crystal for the first time on an island in the Red Sea upon which they landed. It was named by them, as was the beautiful stone they discovered there, as topazos, being the Arabic for something akin to "sought and found".

However, according to other sources, the name is supposed to be derived from the ancient Hindu word tapas, which means "glow".

Throughout history, many healing effects have been attributed to topaz. It was said that if laid on a wound, it staunched bleeding; that it guarded against poisons; that it strengthened the heart and nervous system; and that it stimulated the taste buds. Topaz was known in antiquity as an aid for drunkenness and alcoholism when taken as a powder.

Astrologically, the topaz is seen as a "stone of joy" and "stone of premonition". In Librans, the blue form of topaz is alleged to drive away melancholy and help establish new friendships. Pink topaz may make it easier for Leos to make decisions; and the precious topaz is supposed to bring luck in business affairs to Geminis.

Healing effects: strengthens the heart, stimulates the taste buds and stanches bleeding.

Astrology: Libra; drives away melancholy. Leo (pink); assists in decision-making. Gemini (precious topaz); confers luck in business affairs.

Name: topaz (precious topaz)
Group: -

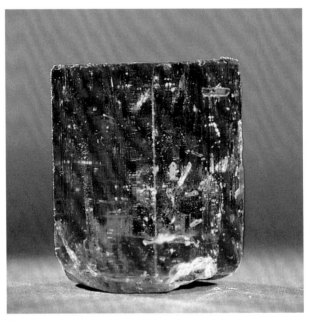

Topaz, Brazil

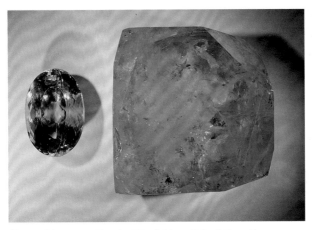

Topaz; blue, raw, Russia (Urals)]; polished, Brazil

Colours: colourless; yellow; reddish brown; light blue; blue; green
Mohs hardness: 8
Specific gravity: 3.49 - 3.6
Crystal system: rhombic
Crystal shape: prismatic, often with multi-facetted
Chemical structure: $Al_2[SiO_4](F, OH)_2$ aluminium silicate containing fluorine
Areas of formation: in pegmatites
Major deposits: Russia (Urals); Namibia; USA; Brazil; Sri Lanka.

TRAPICHE EMERALD

A special crystalline form of emerald, trapiche emerald is found in the Chivor and Muzo mines of Columbia and recently also in Zambia. The crystal form is very characteristic and consists of six sector-like shapes grouped around a centre. This is rather similar to the cross-section through a stem of sugar cane – hence the Spanish name trapiche, which means "little sugar cane mill".

Polished as a cabochon, this configuration is revealed as an embedded, six-pointed star, in the form of fine, black lines.
(See EMERALD for Healing effects and Astrology)

Name: trapiche emerald
Group: beryl group
Colours: emerald green; light green; green; dark green
Mohs hardness: 7.5 - 8
Specific gravity: 2.67 - 2.78
Crystal system: hexagonal
Crystal shape: six-sided prisms in long columns
Chemical structure: $Al_2Be_3[Si_6O_{18}]$ aluminium beryl silicate; green colouration from chromium admixtures
Areas of formation: in hydrothermal gangues
Major deposits: Columbia; Zambia

TURQUOISE

The natural colour of turquoise is reminiscent of that of the sea. This feature made it a sacred stone for the Tibetans, for whom it symbolises the infinity of the sea and the heavens. The Native Americans, especially the Navaho, also prized it highly and still wear it as protection against negative forces.

The Ancient Egyptians, too, knew the turquoise. They discovered rich deposits in the Sinai Peninsula and exploited their finds from very early times.

The name "turquoise" actually derives from "Turkish stone" and would seem to indicate that the gem reached Europe through the returning Crusades - probably after being obtained from Turkish tribes whom they had encountered in Asia Minor.

It almost certainly arrived in Turkey through trade routes with Persia, where the gem was particularly revered at the time of Zoroastra. In this context, the Roman historian, Pliny, recorded that this light green stone was particularly popular as a decorative gem in a part of southern Persia called Carmania, where it was thought to bring luck. Pliny quotes from Al

Kazwini, a Persian scholar as follows: "The hand that wears a turquoise and uses it as a seal will never become poor".

Thus, Persian kings wore turquoise around their necks and on their hands, especially as they believed that the wearer would be protected from sudden, unnatural death. It was also maintained that the gem would become pale when its owner died.

Further east, turquoise was often placed within a frame of pearls and worn on the turban in order to protect the wearer from the "evil eye".

Even as recently as the end of the eighteenth century, turquoise was believed to be fossil teeth or bones that had been affected by strongly colouring substances. It became the popular fashionable gemstone of the "Biedermeier" period in Germany and of the Victorian era in Britain.

In astrology, the turquoise is considered to be the lucky stone of Aquarians, in whom it is said to enhance intuition and independence. It is also worn as a stone of friendship, being believed to ensure fidelity and constancy. It is also reputed to enhance a natural ability to tune in to meditative and healing vibrations.

Healing effects: for throat infections and diseases of the lungs.

Astrology: Aquarius; strengthens the bonds of friendship and encourages creativity.

Name: turquoise (callacite)

Group: -

Colours: sky blue; blue green; turquoise blue

Mohs hardness: 5 – 6

Specific gravity: 2.6 – 2.8

Crystal system: triclinic

Crystal shape: usually grape-bunch-like aggregates

Chemical structure: $CuAl_{16}[(OH)_2/PO_2]_4 \cdot 4H_2O$ alkaline aluminium containing copper

Areas of formation: in clefts of strongly eroded Al_2O_3-rich rocks in association with copper deposits

Major deposits: Poland (Silesia); north-east Iran (Nishapur); USA (Arizona).

TOURMALINE

"The tourmaline is dark,
and what is said there [about it]
is very dark."

Adalbert Stifter, Turmalin

After being almost forgotten, this most colourful of all precious gems was brought back to Europe from Sri Lanka by Dutch seafarers at the beginning of the eighteenth century. Thus, it was practically "rediscovered". One very interesting quality of this gem soon became talked about: the tourmaline builds up a static charge through being rubbed and will then attract small, light particles (such as tobacco ash)– a property that fascinated folks of the time.

Because of its almost unlimited variety of shades of colour, tourmaline soon became another favourite gem of the Biedermeier and mid-Victorian period. During that time, it was also attributed with having secret powers and magical qualities; – and was even believed to maintain chastity.

A reddish variant of tourmaline comes from Siberia and is often called Rubellite – being a derivation from the Latin rubellus, "reddish".

Astrologically, it is assigned to those with the sign of Scorpio and whose "inner fire" is believed to be renewed by the gem. Indigolith is a blue variety of tourmaline and is believed to endow Librans with inner harmony and emotional stability. Green tourmaline is a lucky stone of the sign Capricorn, especially in professional or business matters.

Healing effects: Maintains chastity and general good health; strengthens mental powers.

Astrology: Scorpio (rubellite); maintains "inner fire". Capricorn (indigolith); a lucky stone.

Name: tourmaline (indigolith, rubellite)
Group: tourmaline

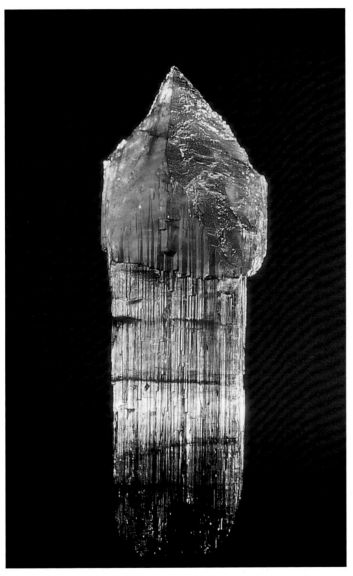

Tourmaline (multi-coloured sceptre crystal), Brazil

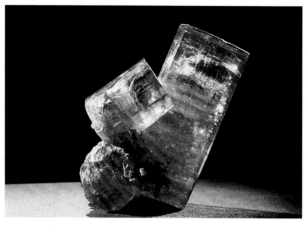

Tourmaline, Brazil

Colours: colourless; pink; brownish; yellow; deep brown; greenish; reddish; violet; polychrome; black

Mohs hardness: 7 – 7.5

Specific gravity: 3.0 – 3.2

Crystal system: trigonal

Crystal shape: usually as longish prisms

Chemical structure: $(Na, Li, Ca) (Fe, Mg, Mn, Al)_3 Al_6 [(OH)_4/(BO_3)_3/Si_6O_{18}]$

Areas of formation: in pegmatites

Major natural deposits: Sri Lanka; Madagascar; Brazil; Mozambique; Angola; USA; Namibia; Pakistan; Afghanistan; Russia.

ZIRCON

Orange-coloured to reddish brown zircons were often called "hyacinths" in earlier times. According to Greek legend, a discus thrown by Apollo killed the young Hyakinthos, and a lily grew up out of his blood. No doubt, it probably seemed appropriate to name a precious gem after a flower.

In magic, the so-called "hyacinth" was highly regarded, as it had the reputation of bringing peace. Whoever wore it was believed to be able to forget previous sorrow and attain an inner contentedness. In the Middle Ages, it was believed that whoever wore a zircon would also be able, in turn, to help another sufferer to attain a similar sense of calm and harmony. Red zircon was also believed to be beneficial to anyone with "diseases of the blood", as it was termed at the time.

In crystal therapy, zircon is used as a tranquillising agent. In astrology, it is assigned to the sign of Taurus and is believed to help a Taurean find spiritual equilibrium and stability.

Healing effects: has a calming effect. Helps with liver and kidney diseases.

Astrology: Taurus; stabilisation of spiritual equilibrium. Leo; a lucky stone. Sagittarius (blue zircon); a protective stone.

Name: zircon
Group: -
Colours: colourless; yellow; red; brown; brown green; blue; pale clove brown
Mohs hardness: 6.5 – 7.5
Specific gravity: 3.90 – 4.71
Crystal system: tetragonal
Crystal shape: short, squat, four-sided prisms
Chemical structure: $Zr[SiO_4]$ zirconium silicate
Areas of formation: typical accompanying mineral in acidic magmatite and metamorphic rocks (granites)
Major deposits: Sri Lanka; Cambodia; Australia; Thailand; Myanmar (Burma); Norway.

The Authors

Andreas Guhr

born 1950 in Hamburg, Germany

1968-71 Studies at the University of Visual Arts, Hamburg
1971   Founding of MINERALIEN ZENTRUM Andreas Guhr, GmbH
1979   Founding of the Hamburg Mineral Fair (Hamburger Mineralientage)
1986   Co-responsible founder of the DMF-International
1989-93 Solely responsible for the conceptualisation, design and exhibition
         goods for the private museum of Dr. Kashiwagi, Tokyo
1992   Responsible Leader and organizer of the first German-Mongolian
         paleontological expedition to the Gobi desert in cooperation
         with GEO magazine.
1995   Author of »Mythos der Steine«, Ellert und Richter, Hamburg
1998   Founding of the ESGS (European Society of Geological Services), an
         enterprise for planning and executing excavation- and expedition
         projects internationally.
2004   Founding of the MIG AG (Mining Investment AG)

Supplier of international museums like:
Houston Museum of Natural Science
American Museum of Natural History, New York
University Museum of the University of Tokyo
National Museum of Natural History, Smithsonian Institute, Washington D. C.

Member of the AAPS (Association of Applied Paleontological Sciences), Utah, USA
Expert for minerals and fossils for the Chamber of Commerce, Hamburg

Jörg Nagler is professor for North American history at the Friedrich-Schiller-University, Jena and has widely published on US social, political and cultural history, especially on subjects such as war and society, immigration, cultural transfers and African American resistance in the age of slavery.

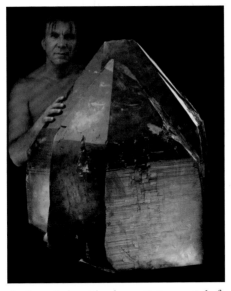

Andreas Guhr with a large citrine crystal of some 660 kg (approx. 1445 lb).

Bibliography

Quote References:

Quotes from *The Epic of Gilgamesh* p. 13 and p. 16, translated by Robert Temple; *He Who Saw Everything* (p. 25, p. 90 and p. 83), Rider Books, London, 1991 used with kind permission of David Higham Associates Ltd.
www.robert-temple.com

Original Work References:

Ägyptisches Totenbuch, Wien 1980

Arthur Beise, *Die Erde*, München o.J.

Friedrich Benesch, *Apokalypse*, Stuttgart 1981

Richard S. Brown (comp.) Austin J. Gordon (ed.), *Handbook of Planetary Gemology*, San Juan Capistrano, Kalifornien 1983

C. W. Ceram, *Götter, Gräber und Gelehrte*, Hamburg 1949

Daya Sarai Chocron, *Heilen mit Edelsteinen*, München 1984

Karl Chudoba/Eduard J. Gübelin, *Edelsteinkundliches Handbuch*, Bonn 1974

Ove Dragsted, *Edelsteine in Farben*, Berlin 1974

W. T. Fernie, *The Occult and Curative Powers of Precious Stones*, San Francisco 1973

Gerda Friess, *Edelsteine im Mittelalter*, Hildesheim 1980

Das Gilgamesch-Epos, Stuttgart 1978

Gerhart Hanslik, *Arzneilich verwendete Mineralien*, Stuttgart 1960

Liselotte Hansmann/Lenz Kriss-Rettenbeck, *Amulett und Talisman*, München 1977

Die Heilige Schrift des Alten und des Neuen Testaments, Zürich 1955

A. Hermann, »Edelsteine«, in: *Reallexikon für Antike und Christentum*, Band 4, 1959

Gertrud I. Hürlimann, *Astrologie*, Schaffhausen 1984

Rudolf Jubelt, *Mineralien*, Leipzig 1976

Friedrich Klockmann, *Lehrbuch der Mineralogie*, Stuttgart 1978

George Frederick Kunz, *The Curious Lore of Precious Stones*, New York 1971

Hans Lüschen, *Die Namen der Steine*, Thun/Schweiz 1979

Michael O'Donoghue, *Enzyklopädie der Minerale und Edelsteine*, Freiburg i. B. 1977

Platon, Sokrates im Gespräch, *Vier Dialoge*, Frankfurt 1960

Wally u. Jenny Richardson/Lenora Huett, *Spiritual Value of Gem Stones*, Marina del Rey/Kalifornien 1984

Peter Riethe (Hg.), *Hildegard von Bingen*, Salzburg 1959

Thomas Ring, *Astrologie ohne Aberglauben*, Düsseldorf 1972

Hans-Jürgen Rösler, *Lehrbuch der Mineralogie*, Leipzig 1981

Julius Ruska, *Das Steinbuch des Pseudo-Aristoteles*, Heidelberg 1912

V. Schloßmacher, *Edelsteine und Perlen*, Stuttgart 1969

Walter Schumann, *Edelsteine und Schmucksteine*, München 1981

Karl Spiesberger, *Magneten des Glücks*, Berlin 1971
Sun Bear & Wabun, *Das Medizinrad*, München 1984
Mellie Uyldert, *Verborgene Kräfte der Edelsteine*, München 1983

Illustration Credits

All photographs by Karl-Christian Lynker, Hamburg, except the following:
Prussian Cultural Collection-Photo-archive: p. 14, 19, 20 (M. Büssing), 21, 33, 35, 39, 41
    43 & 47
Norbert Kustos, Karlsruhe: p. 8-9
Corel: p. 11
Metzeltin Archive, Hamburg: p. 84-85
Monika Ruberg, Hamburg: p. 54-65
South German Picture Library Service: p. 40
University of Hamburg Mineralogical Museum: p. 68, 89, 93, 128, 148 & 154
All used by kind permission of the above sources.

———————————————

Exhibitions of our Earth's Treasures

The 'Steinzeiten' ('Stone Times') exhibition will give you a unique insight into the world of crystals. Here, the emphasis is on experiencing the power of crystals, rather than on the classification and display aspects characteristic of museums. Usually it's only miners who have the privilege of seeing druses (crystal crusts lining caves, and so on); here you too can experience this; or you can journey into the past through gigantic fossil beds; or witness for yourself the power of crystals in meditation rooms. This exhibition will ensure you are touched by your fascinating encounter with crystals.

Steinzeiten, Rödingsmarkt 19
20459 Hamburg, Germany
Tel: +49 40 36900318, Fax: +49 40 36900310
info@steinzeiten.net
www.steinzeiten.net

All the important information about 430 healing gemstones in a neat pocket-book! Michael Gienger, known for his popular introductory work 'Crystal Power, Crystal Healing', here presents a comprehensive directory of all the gemstones currently in use. In a clear, concise and precise style, with pictures accompanying the text, the author describes the characteristics and healing functions of each crystal.

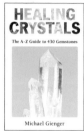

Michael Gienger
Healing Crystals
The A - Z Guide to 430 Gemstones
Paperback, 96 pages
ISBN-13: 978-1-84409-067-9, ISBN 10: 1-84409-067-1

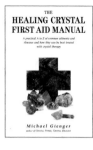

This is an easy-to-use A-Z guide for treating many common ailments and illnesses with the help of crystal therapy. It includes a comprehensive color appendix with photographs and short descriptions of each gemstone recommended.

Michael Gienger
The Healing Crystals First Aid Manual
A Practical A to Z of Common Ailments and Illnesses and How They Can Be Best Treated with Crystal Therapy
288 pages, with 16 colour plates
ISBN-13: 978-1-84409-084-6, ISBN-10: 1-84409-084-1

For further information and book catalogue contact:
Findhorn Press, 305a The Park, Forres IV36 3TE, Scottland.
Earthdancer Books is an Imprint of Findhorn Press.

tel +44 (0)1309-690582   fax +44 (0)1309-690036

info@findhornpress.com www.findhornpress.com www.earthdancer.co.uk

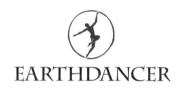

EARTHDANCER

A FINDHORN PRESS IMPRINT